AROMATHERAPY

A MEDICAL DICTIONARY, BIBLIOGRAPHY,
AND ANNOTATED RESEARCH GUIDE TO
INTERNET REFERENCES

JAMES N. PARKER, M.D.
AND PHILIP M. PARKER, PH.D., EDITORS

ii

ICON Health Publications
ICON Group International, Inc.
4370 La Jolla Village Drive, 4th Floor
San Diego, CA 92122 USA

Copyright ©2003 by ICON Group International, Inc.

Copyright ©2003 by ICON Group International, Inc. All rights reserved. This book is protected by copyright. No part of it may be reproduced, stored in a retrieval system, or transmitted in any form or by any means, electronic, mechanical, photocopying, recording, or otherwise, without written permission from the publisher.

Printed in the United States of America.

Last digit indicates print number: 10 9 8 7 6 4 5 3 2 1

Publisher, Health Care: Philip Parker, Ph.D.
Editor(s): James Parker, M.D., Philip Parker, Ph.D.

Publisher's note: The ideas, procedures, and suggestions contained in this book are not intended for the diagnosis or treatment of a health problem. As new medical or scientific information becomes available from academic and clinical research, recommended treatments and drug therapies may undergo changes. The authors, editors, and publisher have attempted to make the information in this book up to date and accurate in accord with accepted standards at the time of publication. The authors, editors, and publisher are not responsible for errors or omissions or for consequences from application of the book, and make no warranty, expressed or implied, in regard to the contents of this book. Any practice described in this book should be applied by the reader in accordance with professional standards of care used in regard to the unique circumstances that may apply in each situation. The reader is advised to always check product information (package inserts) for changes and new information regarding dosage and contraindications before prescribing any drug or pharmacological product. Caution is especially urged when using new or infrequently ordered drugs, herbal remedies, vitamins and supplements, alternative therapies, complementary therapies and medicines, and integrative medical treatments.

Cataloging-in-Publication Data

Parker, James N., 1961-
Parker, Philip M., 1960-

Aromatherapy: A Medical Dictionary, Bibliography, and Annotated Research Guide to Internet References / James N. Parker and Philip M. Parker, editors
           p.   cm.
     Includes bibliographical references, glossary, and index.
     ISBN: 0-597-83587-X
     1. Aromatherapy-Popular works.   I. Title.

Disclaimer

This publication is not intended to be used for the diagnosis or treatment of a health problem. It is sold with the understanding that the publisher, editors, and authors are not engaging in the rendering of medical, psychological, financial, legal, or other professional services.

References to any entity, product, service, or source of information that may be contained in this publication should not be considered an endorsement, either direct or implied, by the publisher, editors, or authors. ICON Group International, Inc., the editors, and the authors are not responsible for the content of any Web pages or publications referenced in this publication.

Copyright Notice

If a physician wishes to copy limited passages from this book for patient use, this right is automatically granted without written permission from ICON Group International, Inc. (ICON Group). However, all of ICON Group publications have copyrights. With exception to the above, copying our publications in whole or in part, for whatever reason, is a violation of copyright laws and can lead to penalties and fines. Should you want to copy tables, graphs, or other materials, please contact us to request permission (E-mail: iconedit@san.rr.com). ICON Group often grants permission for very limited reproduction of our publications for internal use, press releases, and academic research. Such reproduction requires confirmed permission from ICON Group International Inc. **The disclaimer above must accompany all reproductions, in whole or in part, of this book.**

Acknowledgements

The collective knowledge generated from academic and applied research summarized in various references has been critical in the creation of this book which is best viewed as a comprehensive compilation and collection of information prepared by various official agencies which produce publications on aromatherapy. Books in this series draw from various agencies and institutions associated with the United States Department of Health and Human Services, and in particular, the Office of the Secretary of Health and Human Services (OS), the Administration for Children and Families (ACF), the Administration on Aging (AOA), the Agency for Healthcare Research and Quality (AHRQ), the Agency for Toxic Substances and Disease Registry (ATSDR), the Centers for Disease Control and Prevention (CDC), the Food and Drug Administration (FDA), the Healthcare Financing Administration (HCFA), the Health Resources and Services Administration (HRSA), the Indian Health Service (IHS), the institutions of the National Institutes of Health (NIH), the Program Support Center (PSC), and the Substance Abuse and Mental Health Services Administration (SAMHSA). In addition to these sources, information gathered from the National Library of Medicine, the United States Patent Office, the European Union, and their related organizations has been invaluable in the creation of this book. Some of the work represented was financially supported by the Research and Development Committee at INSEAD. This support is gratefully acknowledged. Finally, special thanks are owed to Tiffany Freeman for her excellent editorial support.

About the Editors

James N. Parker, M.D.

Dr. James N. Parker received his Bachelor of Science degree in Psychobiology from the University of California, Riverside and his M.D. from the University of California, San Diego. In addition to authoring numerous research publications, he has lectured at various academic institutions. Dr. Parker is the medical editor for health books by ICON Health Publications.

Philip M. Parker, Ph.D.

Philip M. Parker is the Eli Lilly Chair Professor of Innovation, Business and Society at INSEAD (Fontainebleau, France and Singapore). Dr. Parker has also been Professor at the University of California, San Diego and has taught courses at Harvard University, the Hong Kong University of Science and Technology, the Massachusetts Institute of Technology, Stanford University, and UCLA. Dr. Parker is the associate editor for ICON Health Publications.

About ICON Health Publications

To discover more about ICON Health Publications, simply check with your preferred online booksellers, including Barnes & Noble.com and Amazon.com which currently carry all of our titles. Or, feel free to contact us directly for bulk purchases or institutional discounts:

ICON Group International, Inc.
4370 La Jolla Village Drive, Fourth Floor
San Diego, CA 92122 USA
Fax: 858-546-4341
Web site: **www.icongrouponline.com/health**

Table of Contents

FORWARD

In March 2001, the National Institutes of Health issued the following warning: "The number of Web sites offering health-related resources grows every day. Many sites provide valuable information, while others may have information that is unreliable or misleading."[1] Furthermore, because of the rapid increase in Internet-based information, many hours can be wasted searching, selecting, and printing. Since only the smallest fraction of information dealing with aromatherapy is indexed in search engines, such as **www.google.com** or others, a non-systematic approach to Internet research can be not only time consuming, but also incomplete. This book was created for medical professionals, students, and members of the general public who want to know as much as possible about aromatherapy, using the most advanced research tools available and spending the least amount of time doing so.

In addition to offering a structured and comprehensive bibliography, the pages that follow will tell you where and how to find reliable information covering virtually all topics related to aromatherapy, from the essentials to the most advanced areas of research. Public, academic, government, and peer-reviewed research studies are emphasized. Various abstracts are reproduced to give you some of the latest official information available to date on aromatherapy. Abundant guidance is given on how to obtain free-of-charge primary research results via the Internet. **While this book focuses on the field of medicine, when some sources provide access to non-medical information relating to aromatherapy, these are noted in the text.**

E-book and electronic versions of this book are fully interactive with each of the Internet sites mentioned (clicking on a hyperlink automatically opens your browser to the site indicated). If you are using the hard copy version of this book, you can access a cited Web site by typing the provided Web address directly into your Internet browser. You may find it useful to refer to synonyms or related terms when accessing these Internet databases. **NOTE:** At the time of publication, the Web addresses were functional. However, some links may fail due to URL address changes, which is a common occurrence on the Internet.

For readers unfamiliar with the Internet, detailed instructions are offered on how to access electronic resources. For readers unfamiliar with medical terminology, a comprehensive glossary is provided. For readers without access to Internet resources, a directory of medical libraries, that have or can locate references cited here, is given. We hope these resources will prove useful to the widest possible audience seeking information on aromatherapy.

The Editors

---

[1] From the NIH, National Cancer Institute (NCI): **http://www.cancer.gov/cancerinfo/ten-things-to-know**.

CHAPTER 1. STUDIES ON AROMATHERAPY

Overview

In this chapter, we will show you how to locate peer-reviewed references and studies on aromatherapy.

The Combined Health Information Database

The Combined Health Information Database summarizes studies across numerous federal agencies. To limit your investigation to research studies and aromatherapy, you will need to use the advanced search options. First, go to **http://chid.nih.gov/index.html**. From there, select the "Detailed Search" option (or go directly to that page with the following hyperlink: **http://chid.nih.gov/detail/detail.html**). The trick in extracting studies is found in the drop boxes at the bottom of the search page where "You may refine your search by." Select the dates and language you prefer, and the format option "Journal Article." At the top of the search form, select the number of records you would like to see (we recommend 100) and check the box to display "whole records." We recommend that you type "aromatherapy" (or synonyms) into the "For these words:" box. Consider using the option "anywhere in record" to make your search as broad as possible. If you want to limit the search to only a particular field, such as the title of the journal, then select this option in the "Search in these fields" drop box. The following is what you can expect from this type of search:

- **Use of Aromatherapy as a Complementary Treatment for Chronic Pain**

    Source: Alternative Therapies in Health and Medicine. 5(5): 42-51. September 1999.

    Summary: This article discusses the use of aromatherapy as a complementary treatment for chronic pain. First, it defines aromatherapy, reviews the effects of aroma on the body, and describes methods of using aromatherapy with and without touch. Then, it summarizes human studies on the use of aromatherapy in the treatment of pain, including aromatherapy for children, lavender for pain and coping, chamomile for pain in cancer, marigold for pain in hyperkeratotic plantar lesions, peppermint for headache and arthritic pain, and rose for pain in cancer with bone metastases. Finally, it reviews animal studies, and discusses the potential for untoward effects. It includes a list of essential oils with analgesic properties that are safe to use. The article has 4 tables and 96 references.

- **Single Case Evaluation of the Effects of Aromatherapy and Massage on Disturbed Behaviour in Severe Dementia**

  Source: British Journal of Clinical Psychology. 36: 287-296. 1997.

  Summary: This journal article describes a study of the effects of aromatherapy and massage on disturbed behavior in patients with severe dementia. The participants were four patients on a continuing care ward for people with advanced dementia. Two patients had Alzheimer's disease (AD), one had AD and Parkinson's disease, and one had a frontal lobe disorder. Each participant received 8 to 12 treatment sessions of aromatherapy alone, massage alone, and aromatherapy and massage combined over a 3 month period. Using a single case design with each patient serving as his own control, the effects of each teatment on the patient's behavior was assessed against a no-treatment control condition. The results were mixed. In two patients, all of the treatment conditions decreased disturbed behavior compared with the control condition; however, the effect was significant for only one of these patients. In the other two patients, all or some of the treatment conditions led to an increase in disturbed behavior. The authors discuss possible explanations for the different effects. 4 figures, 1 table, 9 references.

Federally Funded Research on Aromatherapy

The U.S. Government supports a variety of research studies relating to aromatherapy. These studies are tracked by the Office of Extramural Research at the National Institutes of Health.[2] CRISP (Computerized Retrieval of Information on Scientific Projects) is a searchable database of federally funded biomedical research projects conducted at universities, hospitals, and other institutions.

Search the CRISP Web site at **http://crisp.cit.nih.gov/crisp/crisp_query.generate_screen**. You will have the option to perform targeted searches by various criteria, including geography, date, and topics related to aromatherapy.

For most of the studies, the agencies reporting into CRISP provide summaries or abstracts. As opposed to clinical trial research using patients, many federally funded studies use animals or simulated models to explore aromatherapy. The following is typical of the type of information found when searching the CRISP database for aromatherapy:

- **Project Title: AROMATHERAPY & PSYCHOPHYSIOLOGICAL REACTIVITY**

  Principal Investigator & Institution: Sloan, Richard; Columbia University Health Sciences New York, NY 10032

  Timing: Fiscal Year 2001

  Summary: This abstract is not available.

  Website: http://crisp.cit.nih.gov/crisp/Crisp_Query.Generate_Screen

---

[2] Healthcare projects are funded by the National Institutes of Health (NIH), Substance Abuse and Mental Health Services (SAMHSA), Health Resources and Services Administration (HRSA), Food and Drug Administration (FDA), Centers for Disease Control and Prevention (CDCP), Agency for Healthcare Research and Quality (AHRQ), and Office of Assistant Secretary of Health (OASH).

The National Library of Medicine: PubMed

One of the quickest and most comprehensive ways to find academic studies in both English and other languages is to use PubMed, maintained by the National Library of Medicine.[3] The advantage of PubMed over previously mentioned sources is that it covers a greater number of domestic and foreign references. It is also free to use. If the publisher has a Web site that offers full text of its journals, PubMed will provide links to that site, as well as to sites offering other related data. User registration, a subscription fee, or some other type of fee may be required to access the full text of articles in some journals.

To generate your own bibliography of studies dealing with aromatherapy, simply go to the PubMed Web site at **http://www.ncbi.nlm.nih.gov/pubmed**. Type "aromatherapy" (or synonyms) into the search box, and click "Go." The following is the type of output you can expect from PubMed for "aromatherapy" (hyperlinks lead to article summaries):

- **A clinical trial of the effect of aromatherapy on motivational behaviour in a dementia care setting using a single subject design.**
  Author(s): MacMahon S, Kermode S.
  Source: Aust J Holist Nurs. 1998 October; 5(2): 47-9.
  http://www.ncbi.nlm.nih.gov:80/entrez/query.fcgi?cmd=Retrieve&db=PubMed&list_uids=10428895&dopt=Abstract

- **A pilot study addressing the effect of aromatherapy massage on mood, anxiety and relaxation in adult mental health.**
  Author(s): Edge J.
  Source: Complementary Therapies in Nursing & Midwifery. 2003 May; 9(2): 90-7.
  http://www.ncbi.nlm.nih.gov:80/entrez/query.fcgi?cmd=Retrieve&db=PubMed&list_uids=12697161&dopt=Abstract

- **A randomized trial of aromatherapy to reduce anxiety before abortion.**
  Author(s): Wiebe E.
  Source: Effective Clinical Practice : Ecp. 2000 July-August; 3(4): 166-9.
  http://www.ncbi.nlm.nih.gov:80/entrez/query.fcgi?cmd=Retrieve&db=PubMed&list_uids=11183431&dopt=Abstract

- **A review of the literature surrounding the research into aromatherapy.**
  Author(s): Cawthorn A.
  Source: Complementary Therapies in Nursing & Midwifery. 1995 August; 1(4): 118-20. Review.
  http://www.ncbi.nlm.nih.gov:80/entrez/query.fcgi?cmd=Retrieve&db=PubMed&list_uids=9456723&dopt=Abstract

---

[3] PubMed was developed by the National Center for Biotechnology Information (NCBI) at the National Library of Medicine (NLM) at the National Institutes of Health (NIH). The PubMed database was developed in conjunction with publishers of biomedical literature as a search tool for accessing literature citations and linking to full-text journal articles at Web sites of participating publishers. Publishers that participate in PubMed supply NLM with their citations electronically prior to or at the time of publication.

- **Accidental bullous phototoxic reactions to bergamot aromatherapy oil.**
  Author(s): Kaddu S, Kerl H, Wolf P.
  Source: Journal of the American Academy of Dermatology. 2001 September; 45(3): 458-61.
  http://www.ncbi.nlm.nih.gov:80/entrez/query.fcgi?cmd=Retrieve&db=PubMed&list_uids=11511848&dopt=Abstract

- **Advancing my health care practice in aromatherapy.**
  Author(s): Clarke DA.
  Source: Aust J Holist Nurs. 1999 April; 6(1): 32-8.
  http://www.ncbi.nlm.nih.gov:80/entrez/query.fcgi?cmd=Retrieve&db=PubMed&list_uids=11898200&dopt=Abstract

- **Allergic airborne contact dermatitis from essential oils used in aromatherapy.**
  Author(s): Schaller M, Korting HC.
  Source: Clinical and Experimental Dermatology. 1995 March; 20(2): 143-5.
  http://www.ncbi.nlm.nih.gov:80/entrez/query.fcgi?cmd=Retrieve&db=PubMed&list_uids=8565250&dopt=Abstract

- **Allergic contact dermatitis from aromatherapy.**
  Author(s): Weiss RR, James WD.
  Source: American Journal of Contact Dermatitis : Official Journal of the American Contact Dermatitis Society. 1997 December; 8(4): 250-1.
  http://www.ncbi.nlm.nih.gov:80/entrez/query.fcgi?cmd=Retrieve&db=PubMed&list_uids=9358122&dopt=Abstract

- **An evaluation of aromatherapy massage in palliative care.**
  Author(s): Wilkinson S, Aldridge J, Salmon I, Cain E, Wilson B.
  Source: Palliative Medicine. 1999 September; 13(5): 409-17.
  http://www.ncbi.nlm.nih.gov:80/entrez/query.fcgi?cmd=Retrieve&db=PubMed&list_uids=10659113&dopt=Abstract

- **An investigation into the use of aromatherapy in intrapartum midwifery practice.**
  Author(s): Burns EE, Blamey C, Ersser SJ, Barnetson L, Lloyd AJ.
  Source: Journal of Alternative and Complementary Medicine (New York, N.Y.). 2000 April; 6(2): 141-7.
  http://www.ncbi.nlm.nih.gov:80/entrez/query.fcgi?cmd=Retrieve&db=PubMed&list_uids=10784271&dopt=Abstract

- **'Aroma 2000–fragrancing the future'. Favre Armstrong reports on the first Baltic States Aromatherapy Conference.**
  Author(s): Armstrong F.
  Source: Complementary Therapies in Nursing & Midwifery. 2001 May; 7(2): 104-7.
  http://www.ncbi.nlm.nih.gov:80/entrez/query.fcgi?cmd=Retrieve&db=PubMed&list_uids=11855769&dopt=Abstract

- **Aromatherapy again.**
  Author(s): Vickers A.
  Source: The British Journal of General Practice : the Journal of the Royal College of General Practitioners. 2000 November; 50(460): 920.
  http://www.ncbi.nlm.nih.gov:80/entrez/query.fcgi?cmd=Retrieve&db=PubMed&list_uids=11141888&dopt=Abstract

- **Aromatherapy and behaviour disturbances in dementia: a randomized controlled trial.**
  Author(s): Smallwood J, Brown R, Coulter F, Irvine E, Copland C.
  Source: International Journal of Geriatric Psychiatry. 2001 October; 16(10): 1010-3.
  http://www.ncbi.nlm.nih.gov:80/entrez/query.fcgi?cmd=Retrieve&db=PubMed&list_uids=11607948&dopt=Abstract

- **Aromatherapy and its application in cancer and palliative care.**
  Author(s): Cawthorn A, Carter A.
  Source: Complementary Therapies in Nursing & Midwifery. 2000 May; 6(2): 83-6.
  http://www.ncbi.nlm.nih.gov:80/entrez/query.fcgi?cmd=Retrieve&db=PubMed&list_uids=10844746&dopt=Abstract

- **Aromatherapy and its application in the management of people with dementia.**
  Author(s): Tobin P.
  Source: Lamp. 1995 June; 52(5): 34. No Abstract Available.
  http://www.ncbi.nlm.nih.gov:80/entrez/query.fcgi?cmd=Retrieve&db=PubMed&list_uids=7500733&dopt=Abstract

- **Aromatherapy and massage.**
  Author(s): Hanse M.
  Source: Nursing Standard : Official Newspaper of the Royal College of Nursing. 1990 August 22-28; 4(48): 43.
  http://www.ncbi.nlm.nih.gov:80/entrez/query.fcgi?cmd=Retrieve&db=PubMed&list_uids=2169854&dopt=Abstract

- **Aromatherapy and massage: the evidence.**
  Author(s): Buckle S.
  Source: Paediatric Nursing. 2003 July; 15(6): 24-7. Review.
  http://www.ncbi.nlm.nih.gov:80/entrez/query.fcgi?cmd=Retrieve&db=PubMed&list_uids=12889317&dopt=Abstract

- **Aromatherapy and the use of scents in psychotherapy.**
  Author(s): La Torre MA.
  Source: Perspectives in Psychiatric Care. 2003 January-March; 39(1): 35-7.
  http://www.ncbi.nlm.nih.gov:80/entrez/query.fcgi?cmd=Retrieve&db=PubMed&list_uids=12724965&dopt=Abstract

- **Aromatherapy as a safe and effective treatment for the management of agitation in severe dementia: the results of a double-blind, placebo-controlled trial with Melissa.**
  Author(s): Ballard CG, O'Brien JT, Reichelt K, Perry EK.
  Source: The Journal of Clinical Psychiatry. 2002 July; 63(7): 553-8.
  http://www.ncbi.nlm.nih.gov:80/entrez/query.fcgi?cmd=Retrieve&db=PubMed&list_uids=12143909&dopt=Abstract

- **Aromatherapy as an adjunct to care in a mental health day hospital.**
  Author(s): Hicks G.
  Source: Journal of Psychiatric and Mental Health Nursing. 1998 August; 5(4): 317.
  http://www.ncbi.nlm.nih.gov:80/entrez/query.fcgi?cmd=Retrieve&db=PubMed&list_uids=9807369&dopt=Abstract

- **Aromatherapy for deaf and deafblind people living in residential accommodation.**
  Author(s): Armstrong F, Heidingsfeld V.
  Source: Complementary Therapies in Nursing & Midwifery. 2000 November; 6(4): 180-8.
  http://www.ncbi.nlm.nih.gov:80/entrez/query.fcgi?cmd=Retrieve&db=PubMed&list_uids=11858301&dopt=Abstract

- **Aromatherapy for Health Professionals annual report.**
  Author(s): Buckle J.
  Source: Beginnings. 2001 January-February; 21(1): 9, 12. No Abstract Available.
  http://www.ncbi.nlm.nih.gov:80/entrez/query.fcgi?cmd=Retrieve&db=PubMed&list_uids=11898298&dopt=Abstract

- **Aromatherapy for health professionals.**
  Author(s): Buckle J.
  Source: Beginnings. 2003 January-February; 23(1): 6-7. No Abstract Available.
  http://www.ncbi.nlm.nih.gov:80/entrez/query.fcgi?cmd=Retrieve&db=PubMed&list_uids=12592972&dopt=Abstract

- **Aromatherapy for health professionals.**
  Author(s): Waterworth S.
  Source: Australian Nursing Journal (July 1993). 1999 September; 7(3): 37.
  http://www.ncbi.nlm.nih.gov:80/entrez/query.fcgi?cmd=Retrieve&db=PubMed&list_uids=11894265&dopt=Abstract

- **Aromatherapy for health professionals.**
  Author(s): Buckle J.
  Source: Beginnings. 2002 January-February; 22(1): 7. No Abstract Available.
  http://www.ncbi.nlm.nih.gov:80/entrez/query.fcgi?cmd=Retrieve&db=PubMed&list_uids=11842643&dopt=Abstract

- **Aromatherapy growing rapidly.**
  Author(s): Belcher I.
  Source: Beginnings. 1996 February; 16(2): 4. No Abstract Available.
  http://www.ncbi.nlm.nih.gov:80/entrez/query.fcgi?cmd=Retrieve&db=PubMed&list_uids=8704372&dopt=Abstract

- **Aromatherapy in arthritis: a study.**
  Author(s): Brownfield A.
  Source: Nursing Standard : Official Newspaper of the Royal College of Nursing. 1998 October 21-27; 13(5): 34-5.
  http://www.ncbi.nlm.nih.gov:80/entrez/query.fcgi?cmd=Retrieve&db=PubMed&list_uids=9919184&dopt=Abstract

- **Aromatherapy in dermatology.**
  Author(s): Stevensen CJ.
  Source: Clinics in Dermatology. 1998 November-December; 16(6): 689-94. Review.
  http://www.ncbi.nlm.nih.gov:80/entrez/query.fcgi?cmd=Retrieve&db=PubMed&list_uids=9949913&dopt=Abstract

- **Aromatherapy in midwifery: benefits and risks.**
  Author(s): Tiran D.
  Source: Complementary Therapies in Nursing & Midwifery. 1996 August; 2(4): 88-92. Review.
  http://www.ncbi.nlm.nih.gov:80/entrez/query.fcgi?cmd=Retrieve&db=PubMed&list_uids=9439282&dopt=Abstract

- **Aromatherapy in perianesthesia nursing.**
  Author(s): Buckle J.
  Source: Journal of Perianesthesia Nursing : Official Journal of the American Society of Perianesthesia Nurses / American Society of Perianesthesia Nurses. 1999 December; 14(6): 336-44. Review.
  http://www.ncbi.nlm.nih.gov:80/entrez/query.fcgi?cmd=Retrieve&db=PubMed&list_uids=10839071&dopt=Abstract

- **Aromatherapy in practice.**
  Author(s): Avis A.
  Source: Nursing Standard : Official Newspaper of the Royal College of Nursing. 1999 March 3-9; 13(24): 14-5.
  http://www.ncbi.nlm.nih.gov:80/entrez/query.fcgi?cmd=Retrieve&db=PubMed&list_uids=10335230&dopt=Abstract

- **Aromatherapy in practice: creative nursing care--Daw House Hospice.**
  Author(s): Osborne R.
  Source: Aust J Holist Nurs. 1998 October; 5(2): 50. No Abstract Available.
  http://www.ncbi.nlm.nih.gov:80/entrez/query.fcgi?cmd=Retrieve&db=PubMed&list_uids=10428896&dopt=Abstract

- **Aromatherapy in the care of older people.**
  Author(s): Brett H.
  Source: Nurs Times. 1999 August 18-24; 95(33): 56-7. No Abstract Available.
  http://www.ncbi.nlm.nih.gov:80/entrez/query.fcgi?cmd=Retrieve&db=PubMed&list_uids=10614423&dopt=Abstract

- **Aromatherapy massage for joint pain and constipation in a patient with Guillian Barre.**
  Author(s): Shirreffs CM.
  Source: Complementary Therapies in Nursing & Midwifery. 2001 May; 7(2): 78-83.
  http://www.ncbi.nlm.nih.gov:80/entrez/query.fcgi?cmd=Retrieve&db=PubMed&list_uids=11855776&dopt=Abstract

- **Aromatherapy massage: its use in a ward setting.**
  Author(s): Mullins P.
  Source: Nurs Times. 2002 May 28-June 3; 98(22): 36-7. Review.
  http://www.ncbi.nlm.nih.gov:80/entrez/query.fcgi?cmd=Retrieve&db=PubMed&list_uids=12168454&dopt=Abstract

- **Aromatherapy positively affects mood, EEG patterns of alertness and math computations.**
  Author(s): Diego MA, Jones NA, Field T, Hernandez-Reif M, Schanberg S, Kuhn C, McAdam V, Galamaga R, Galamaga M.
  Source: The International Journal of Neuroscience. 1998 December; 96(3-4): 217-24.
  http://www.ncbi.nlm.nih.gov:80/entrez/query.fcgi?cmd=Retrieve&db=PubMed&list_uids=10069621&dopt=Abstract

- **Aromatherapy.**
  Author(s): Eliopoulos C.
  Source: Director. 1999 Autumn; 7(4): 132. No Abstract Available.
  http://www.ncbi.nlm.nih.gov:80/entrez/query.fcgi?cmd=Retrieve&db=PubMed&list_uids=10703342&dopt=Abstract

- **Aromatherapy.**
  Author(s): Trevelyan J.
  Source: Nurs Times. 1993 June 23-29; 89(25): 38-40. No Abstract Available.
  http://www.ncbi.nlm.nih.gov:80/entrez/query.fcgi?cmd=Retrieve&db=PubMed&list_uids=8321693&dopt=Abstract

- **Aromatherapy.**
  Author(s): Buckle J.
  Source: Nurs Times. 1993 May 19-25; 89(20): 32-5.
  http://www.ncbi.nlm.nih.gov:80/entrez/query.fcgi?cmd=Retrieve&db=PubMed&list_uids=8321672&dopt=Abstract

- **Aromatherapy.**
  Author(s): Armstrong F.
  Source: Prof Nurse. 1986 August; 1(11): 305. No Abstract Available.
  http://www.ncbi.nlm.nih.gov:80/entrez/query.fcgi?cmd=Retrieve&db=PubMed&list_uids=3638730&dopt=Abstract

- **Aromatherapy. Introduction into a maternity service.**
  Author(s): Jardine M.
  Source: Pract Midwife. 2002 April; 5(4): 14-5. No Abstract Available.
  http://www.ncbi.nlm.nih.gov:80/entrez/query.fcgi?cmd=Retrieve&db=PubMed&list_
  uids=11987879&dopt=Abstract

- **Aromatherapy. Working with clients who are HIV positive.**
  Author(s): Toomer S.
  Source: Nursing Standard : Official Newspaper of the Royal College of Nursing. 1994
  April 20-26; 8(30): 83.
  http://www.ncbi.nlm.nih.gov:80/entrez/query.fcgi?cmd=Retrieve&db=PubMed&list_
  uids=8003428&dopt=Abstract

- **Aromatherapy: a matter for debate.**
  Author(s): Hobbs S.
  Source: Complementary Therapies in Nursing & Midwifery. 1997 December; 3(6): 171.
  http://www.ncbi.nlm.nih.gov:80/entrez/query.fcgi?cmd=Retrieve&db=PubMed&list_
  uids=9511648&dopt=Abstract

- **Aromatherapy: a survey of current practice in the management of rheumatic disease symptoms.**
  Author(s): Osborn CE, Barlas P, Baxter GD, Barlow JH.
  Source: Complementary Therapies in Medicine. 2001 June; 9(2): 62-7.
  http://www.ncbi.nlm.nih.gov:80/entrez/query.fcgi?cmd=Retrieve&db=PubMed&list_
  uids=11444884&dopt=Abstract

- **Aromatherapy: a systematic review.**
  Author(s): Cooke B, Ernst E.
  Source: The British Journal of General Practice : the Journal of the Royal College of
  General Practitioners. 2000 June; 50(455): 493-6. Review.
  http://www.ncbi.nlm.nih.gov:80/entrez/query.fcgi?cmd=Retrieve&db=PubMed&list_
  uids=10962794&dopt=Abstract

- **Aromatherapy: ineffective treatment or effective placebo?**
  Author(s): Bent S.
  Source: Effective Clinical Practice : Ecp. 2000 July-August; 3(4): 188-90.
  http://www.ncbi.nlm.nih.gov:80/entrez/query.fcgi?cmd=Retrieve&db=PubMed&list_
  uids=11183435&dopt=Abstract

- **Aromatherapy: is it for real?**
  Author(s): Cerrato PL.
  Source: Rn. 1998 June; 61(6): 51-2. Review.
  http://www.ncbi.nlm.nih.gov:80/entrez/query.fcgi?cmd=Retrieve&db=PubMed&list_
  uids=9668906&dopt=Abstract

- **Aromatherapy: mythical, magical, or medicinal?**
  Author(s): Thomas DV.
  Source: Holistic Nursing Practice. 2002 October; 16(5): 8-16. Review.
  http://www.ncbi.nlm.nih.gov:80/entrez/query.fcgi?cmd=Retrieve&db=PubMed&list_
  uids=12465213&dopt=Abstract

- **Aromatherapy: the essentials (continuing education credit).**
  Author(s): Stevenson C.
  Source: Nursing Standard : Official Newspaper of the Royal College of Nursing. 1994
  November 23-29; 9(9 Suppl Nu): 3-8; Quiz 11-3.
  http://www.ncbi.nlm.nih.gov:80/entrez/query.fcgi?cmd=Retrieve&db=PubMed&list_
  uids=7811632&dopt=Abstract

- **Aromatherapy: the scents for survival.**
  Author(s): Buckle J.
  Source: Beginnings. 1994 May; 14(5): 1, 7. No Abstract Available.
  http://www.ncbi.nlm.nih.gov:80/entrez/query.fcgi?cmd=Retrieve&db=PubMed&list_
  uids=7795337&dopt=Abstract

- **Aromatherapy: the smell of success. Interview by Jackie O'Byrne.**
  Author(s): Clifford F.
  Source: Nursing Standard : Official Newspaper of the Royal College of Nursing. 1990
  August 15-21; 4(47): 23.
  http://www.ncbi.nlm.nih.gov:80/entrez/query.fcgi?cmd=Retrieve&db=PubMed&list_
  uids=2169853&dopt=Abstract

- **Aromatherapy: therapeutic applications of plant essential oils.**
  Author(s): Halcon LL.
  Source: Minn Med. 2002 November; 85(11): 42-6.
  http://www.ncbi.nlm.nih.gov:80/entrez/query.fcgi?cmd=Retrieve&db=PubMed&list_
  uids=12498066&dopt=Abstract

- **Aromatherapy—nice but not 'essential'.**
  Author(s): Mackereth P.
  Source: Complementary Therapies in Nursing & Midwifery. 1995 February; 1(1): 47.
  Review.
  http://www.ncbi.nlm.nih.gov:80/entrez/query.fcgi?cmd=Retrieve&db=PubMed&list_
  uids=9456699&dopt=Abstract

- **Can aromatherapy replace pre-medication?**
  Author(s): Gibbons E.
  Source: Br J Theatre Nurs. 1998 August; 8(5): 34-6. Review.
  http://www.ncbi.nlm.nih.gov:80/entrez/query.fcgi?cmd=Retrieve&db=PubMed&list_
  uids=9782829&dopt=Abstract

- **Cancer patients' experiences and evaluations of aromatherapy massage in palliative care.**
  Author(s): Dunwoody L, Smyth A, Davidson R.
  Source: International Journal of Palliative Nursing. 2002 October; 8(10): 497-504.
  http://www.ncbi.nlm.nih.gov:80/entrez/query.fcgi?cmd=Retrieve&db=PubMed&list_uids=12419989&dopt=Abstract

- **Clinical aromatherapy and AIDS.**
  Author(s): Buckle J.
  Source: The Journal of the Association of Nurses in Aids Care : Janac. 2002 May-June; 13(3): 81-99.
  http://www.ncbi.nlm.nih.gov:80/entrez/query.fcgi?cmd=Retrieve&db=PubMed&list_uids=12064023&dopt=Abstract

- **Clinical aromatherapy and touch: complementary therapies for nursing practice.**
  Author(s): Buckle J.
  Source: Critical Care Nurse. 1998 October; 18(5): 54-61. Review.
  http://www.ncbi.nlm.nih.gov:80/entrez/query.fcgi?cmd=Retrieve&db=PubMed&list_uids=9934050&dopt=Abstract

- **Clinical aromatherapy. Therapeutic uses for essential oils.**
  Author(s): Buckle J.
  Source: Adv Nurse Pract. 2002 May; 10(5): 67-8, 88. Review. No Abstract Available.
  http://www.ncbi.nlm.nih.gov:80/entrez/query.fcgi?cmd=Retrieve&db=PubMed&list_uids=12420533&dopt=Abstract

- **Complementary medicine. Aromatherapy.**
  Author(s): Trevelyan J, Booth B.
  Source: Nurs Times. 1994 September 21-27; 90(38): Suppl 1-16. No Abstract Available.
  http://www.ncbi.nlm.nih.gov:80/entrez/query.fcgi?cmd=Retrieve&db=PubMed&list_uids=7971321&dopt=Abstract

- **Complementary medicine. Using aromatherapy in childbirth.**
  Author(s): Burns E, Blamey C.
  Source: Nurs Times. 1994 March 2-8; 90(9): 54-60. No Abstract Available.
  http://www.ncbi.nlm.nih.gov:80/entrez/query.fcgi?cmd=Retrieve&db=PubMed&list_uids=8152975&dopt=Abstract

- **Complementary therapies in nursing. Implications for practice using aromatherapy as an example.**
  Author(s): Johnson GR.
  Source: Complementary Therapies in Nursing & Midwifery. 1995 October; 1(5): 128-32. Review.
  http://www.ncbi.nlm.nih.gov:80/entrez/query.fcgi?cmd=Retrieve&db=PubMed&list_uids=9456726&dopt=Abstract

- **Complementary therapy: aromatherapy with massage for geriatric and hospice care--a call for an holistic approach.**
  Author(s): Howdyshell C.
  Source: Hosp J. 1998; 13(3): 69-75. Review.
  http://www.ncbi.nlm.nih.gov:80/entrez/query.fcgi?cmd=Retrieve&db=PubMed&list_uids=9677958&dopt=Abstract

- **Contemporary therapy: aromatherapy in the management of acute pain?**
  Author(s): Ching M.
  Source: Contemp Nurse. 1999 December; 8(4): 146-51.
  http://www.ncbi.nlm.nih.gov:80/entrez/query.fcgi?cmd=Retrieve&db=PubMed&list_uids=11141786&dopt=Abstract

- **Development of an aromatherapy service at a Cancer Centre.**
  Author(s): Kite SM, Maher EJ, Anderson K, Young T, Young J, Wood J, Howells N, Bradburn J.
  Source: Palliative Medicine. 1998 May; 12(3): 171-80.
  http://www.ncbi.nlm.nih.gov:80/entrez/query.fcgi?cmd=Retrieve&db=PubMed&list_uids=9743836&dopt=Abstract

- **Down to basics: the question of base gels and creams for aromatherapy. Interview by Caroline Stevensen.**
  Author(s): Kusmirek J.
  Source: Complementary Therapies in Nursing & Midwifery. 1998 August; 4(4): 118-9.
  http://www.ncbi.nlm.nih.gov:80/entrez/query.fcgi?cmd=Retrieve&db=PubMed&list_uids=9830939&dopt=Abstract

- **Enhancing care using aromatherapy.**
  Author(s): Spurling S.
  Source: Br J Theatre Nurs. 1998 July; 8(4): 36-8. Review. No Abstract Available.
  http://www.ncbi.nlm.nih.gov:80/entrez/query.fcgi?cmd=Retrieve&db=PubMed&list_uids=9782820&dopt=Abstract

- **Essential oils and 'aromatherapy': their modern role in healing.**
  Author(s): Lis-Balchin M.
  Source: J R Soc Health. 1997 October; 117(5): 324-9. Review.
  http://www.ncbi.nlm.nih.gov:80/entrez/query.fcgi?cmd=Retrieve&db=PubMed&list_uids=9519666&dopt=Abstract

- **Evaluation and attributional analysis of an aromatherapy service for older adults with physical health problems and carers using the service.**
  Author(s): Papadopoulos A, Wright S, Ensor J.
  Source: Complementary Therapies in Medicine. 1999 December; 7(4): 239-44.
  http://www.ncbi.nlm.nih.gov:80/entrez/query.fcgi?cmd=Retrieve&db=PubMed&list_uids=10709309&dopt=Abstract

- **Experiences with aromatherapy in the elderly.**
  Author(s): O'Brien B.
  Source: Journal of Alternative and Complementary Medicine (New York, N.Y.). 1997 Fall; 3(3): 211.
  http://www.ncbi.nlm.nih.gov:80/entrez/query.fcgi?cmd=Retrieve&db=PubMed&list_uids=9430321&dopt=Abstract

- **Formation and development of the Aromatherapy Organisations Council.**
  Author(s): Baker S.
  Source: Complementary Therapies in Nursing & Midwifery. 1997 June; 3(3): 77-80.
  http://www.ncbi.nlm.nih.gov:80/entrez/query.fcgi?cmd=Retrieve&db=PubMed&list_uids=9439254&dopt=Abstract

- **Holistic aromatherapy.**
  Author(s): Pounds L.
  Source: Beginnings. 1992 March; 12(3): 1, 4. No Abstract Available.
  http://www.ncbi.nlm.nih.gov:80/entrez/query.fcgi?cmd=Retrieve&db=PubMed&list_uids=1551007&dopt=Abstract

- **Implementing aromatherapy in nursing and midwifery practice.**
  Author(s): Rawlings F, Meerabeau L.
  Source: Journal of Clinical Nursing. 2003 May; 12(3): 405-11.
  http://www.ncbi.nlm.nih.gov:80/entrez/query.fcgi?cmd=Retrieve&db=PubMed&list_uids=12709115&dopt=Abstract

- **Influence of aromatherapy on medication administration to residential-care residents with dementia and behavioral challenges.**
  Author(s): Gray SG, Clair AA.
  Source: Am J Alzheimers Dis Other Demen. 2002 May-June; 17(3): 169-74.
  http://www.ncbi.nlm.nih.gov:80/entrez/query.fcgi?cmd=Retrieve&db=PubMed&list_uids=12083347&dopt=Abstract

- **Inhalation aromatherapy during radiotherapy: results of a placebo-controlled double-blind randomized trial.**
  Author(s): Graham PH, Browne L, Cox H, Graham J.
  Source: Journal of Clinical Oncology : Official Journal of the American Society of Clinical Oncology. 2003 June 15; 21(12): 2372-6.
  http://www.ncbi.nlm.nih.gov:80/entrez/query.fcgi?cmd=Retrieve&db=PubMed&list_uids=12805340&dopt=Abstract

- **Lavender aromatherapy in recovery from exercise.**
  Author(s): Romine IJ, Bush AM, Geist CR.
  Source: Percept Mot Skills. 1999 June; 88(3 Pt 1): 756-8.
  http://www.ncbi.nlm.nih.gov:80/entrez/query.fcgi?cmd=Retrieve&db=PubMed&list_uids=10407881&dopt=Abstract

- **Massage and aromatherapy massage: nursing art and science.**
  Author(s): Buckley J.
  Source: International Journal of Palliative Nursing. 2002 June; 8(6): 276-80. Review.
  http://www.ncbi.nlm.nih.gov:80/entrez/query.fcgi?cmd=Retrieve&db=PubMed&list_uids=12131821&dopt=Abstract

- **Massage and aromatherapy on a leukaemia unit.**
  Author(s): Stringer J.
  Source: Complementary Therapies in Nursing & Midwifery. 2000 May; 6(2): 72-6.
  http://www.ncbi.nlm.nih.gov:80/entrez/query.fcgi?cmd=Retrieve&db=PubMed&list_uids=10844744&dopt=Abstract

- **Measuring the effects of aromatherapy.**
  Author(s): Stevenson C.
  Source: Nurs Times. 1992 October 7-13; 88(41): 62-3. No Abstract Available.
  http://www.ncbi.nlm.nih.gov:80/entrez/query.fcgi?cmd=Retrieve&db=PubMed&list_uids=1491983&dopt=Abstract

- **Patients' views on the factors which would influence the use of an aromatherapy massage out-patient service.**
  Author(s): Kacperek L.
  Source: Complementary Therapies in Nursing & Midwifery. 1997 April; 3(2): 51-7.
  http://www.ncbi.nlm.nih.gov:80/entrez/query.fcgi?cmd=Retrieve&db=PubMed&list_uids=9432431&dopt=Abstract

- **Phototoxic contact dermatitis from 5-methoxypsoralen in aromatherapy oil.**
  Author(s): Clark SM, Wilkinson SM.
  Source: Contact Dermatitis. 1998 May; 38(5): 289-90.
  http://www.ncbi.nlm.nih.gov:80/entrez/query.fcgi?cmd=Retrieve&db=PubMed&list_uids=9667455&dopt=Abstract

- **Possible health and safety problems in the use of novel plant essential oils and extracts in aromatherapy.**
  Author(s): Lis-Balchin M.
  Source: J R Soc Health. 1999 December; 119(4): 240-3. Review.
  http://www.ncbi.nlm.nih.gov:80/entrez/query.fcgi?cmd=Retrieve&db=PubMed&list_uids=10673845&dopt=Abstract

- **Psychological effects of aromatherapy on chronic hemodialysis patients.**
  Author(s): Itai T, Amayasu H, Kuribayashi M, Kawamura N, Okada M, Momose A, Tateyama T, Narumi K, Uematsu W, Kaneko S.
  Source: Psychiatry and Clinical Neurosciences. 2000 August; 54(4): 393-7.
  http://www.ncbi.nlm.nih.gov:80/entrez/query.fcgi?cmd=Retrieve&db=PubMed&list_uids=10997854&dopt=Abstract

- **Randomized trial of aromatherapy. Successful treatment for alopecia areata.**
  Author(s): Hay IC, Jamieson M, Ormerod AD.
  Source: Archives of Dermatology. 1998 November; 134(11): 1349-52.
  http://www.ncbi.nlm.nih.gov:80/entrez/query.fcgi?cmd=Retrieve&db=PubMed&list_uids=9828867&dopt=Abstract

- **Randomized trial of aromatherapy: successful treatment for alopecia areata.**
  Author(s): Kalish RS.
  Source: Archives of Dermatology. 1999 May; 135(5): 602-3.
  http://www.ncbi.nlm.nih.gov:80/entrez/query.fcgi?cmd=Retrieve&db=PubMed&list_uids=10328210&dopt=Abstract

- **Re: Essential oils and 'aromatherapy' their modern role in healing.**
  Author(s): Lis-Balchin M.
  Source: J R Soc Health. 1998 April; 118(2): 126. No Abstract Available.
  http://www.ncbi.nlm.nih.gov:80/entrez/query.fcgi?cmd=Retrieve&db=PubMed&list_uids=10076647&dopt=Abstract

- **Re: Essential oils and 'aromatherapy': their role in healing.**
  Author(s): Packham CL.
  Source: J R Soc Health. 1997 December; 117(6): 400. No Abstract Available.
  http://www.ncbi.nlm.nih.gov:80/entrez/query.fcgi?cmd=Retrieve&db=PubMed&list_uids=9519679&dopt=Abstract

- **Safe practice and aromatherapy.**
  Author(s): Maddocks W.
  Source: Nurs N Z. 1995 November; 1(10): 15-6. No Abstract Available.
  http://www.ncbi.nlm.nih.gov:80/entrez/query.fcgi?cmd=Retrieve&db=PubMed&list_uids=8536097&dopt=Abstract

- **Scientific status of aromatherapy.**
  Author(s): King JR.
  Source: Perspectives in Biology and Medicine. 1994 Spring; 37(3): 409-15.
  http://www.ncbi.nlm.nih.gov:80/entrez/query.fcgi?cmd=Retrieve&db=PubMed&list_uids=8202345&dopt=Abstract

- **Sensing an improvement: an experimental study to evaluate the use of aromatherapy, massage and periods of rest in an intensive care unit.**
  Author(s): Dunn C, Sleep J, Collett D.
  Source: Journal of Advanced Nursing. 1995 January; 21(1): 34-40.
  http://www.ncbi.nlm.nih.gov:80/entrez/query.fcgi?cmd=Retrieve&db=PubMed&list_uids=7897075&dopt=Abstract

- **Should there be aromatherapy for addiction?**
  Author(s): Miller WR, Walker DD.
  Source: Addiction (Abingdon, England). 1997 April; 92(4): 486-7.
  http://www.ncbi.nlm.nih.gov:80/entrez/query.fcgi?cmd=Retrieve&db=PubMed&list_uids=9177073&dopt=Abstract

- **Single case evaluation of the effects of aromatherapy and massage on disturbed behaviour in severe dementia.**
  Author(s): Brooker DJ, Snape M, Johnson E, Ward D, Payne M.
  Source: The British Journal of Clinical Psychology / the British Psychological Society. 1997 May; 36 (Pt 2): 287-96.
  http://www.ncbi.nlm.nih.gov:80/entrez/query.fcgi?cmd=Retrieve&db=PubMed&list_uids=9167869&dopt=Abstract

- **The clinical use of aromatherapy in the reduction of stress.**
  Author(s): Rimmer L.
  Source: Home Healthcare Nurse. 1998 February; 16(2): 123-6.
  http://www.ncbi.nlm.nih.gov:80/entrez/query.fcgi?cmd=Retrieve&db=PubMed&list_uids=9526345&dopt=Abstract

- **The development of clinical practice guidelines for the use of aromatherapy in a cancer setting.**
  Author(s): Campbell L, Pollard A, Roeton C.
  Source: Aust J Holist Nurs. 2001 April; 8(1): 14-22. Review.
  http://www.ncbi.nlm.nih.gov:80/entrez/query.fcgi?cmd=Retrieve&db=PubMed&list_uids=11898289&dopt=Abstract

- **The effect of aromatherapy in promoting relaxation and stress reduction in a general hospital.**
  Author(s): Cannard G.
  Source: Complementary Therapies in Nursing & Midwifery. 1996 April; 2(2): 38-40.
  http://www.ncbi.nlm.nih.gov:80/entrez/query.fcgi?cmd=Retrieve&db=PubMed&list_uids=9439271&dopt=Abstract

- **The effects of aromatherapy on pruritus in patients undergoing hemodialysis.**
  Author(s): Ro YJ, Ha HC, Kim CG, Yeom HA.
  Source: Dermatology Nursing / Dermatology Nurses' Association. 2002 August; 14(4): 231-4, 237-8, 256; Quiz 239.
  http://www.ncbi.nlm.nih.gov:80/entrez/query.fcgi?cmd=Retrieve&db=PubMed&list_uids=12240499&dopt=Abstract

- **The essence of aromatherapy.**
  Author(s): West B.
  Source: Elder Care. 1993 July-August; 5(4): 24-5. No Abstract Available.
  http://www.ncbi.nlm.nih.gov:80/entrez/query.fcgi?cmd=Retrieve&db=PubMed&list_uids=8348128&dopt=Abstract

- **The promise of aromatherapy. Essential oils have been shown in clinical trials to soothe some chronic ills brought on by old age.**
  Author(s): Wood K.
  Source: Provider. 2003 March; 29(3): 47-8. No Abstract Available.
  http://www.ncbi.nlm.nih.gov:80/entrez/query.fcgi?cmd=Retrieve&db=PubMed&list_uids=12666332&dopt=Abstract

- **The role of aromatherapy in nursing care.**
  Author(s): Buckle J.
  Source: Nurs Clin North Am. 2001 March; 36(1): 57-72. Review.
  http://www.ncbi.nlm.nih.gov:80/entrez/query.fcgi?cmd=Retrieve&db=PubMed&list_
  uids=11342402&dopt=Abstract

- **The role of aromatherapy massage in reducing anxiety in patients with malignant brain tumours.**
  Author(s): Hadfield N.
  Source: International Journal of Palliative Nursing. 2001 June; 7(6): 279-85. Review.
  http://www.ncbi.nlm.nih.gov:80/entrez/query.fcgi?cmd=Retrieve&db=PubMed&list_
  uids=12066022&dopt=Abstract

- **The science and art of aromatherapy.**
  Author(s): Robins JL.
  Source: Journal of Holistic Nursing : Official Journal of the American Holistic Nurses' Association. 1999 March; 17(1): 5-17. Review.
  http://www.ncbi.nlm.nih.gov:80/entrez/query.fcgi?cmd=Retrieve&db=PubMed&list_
  uids=10373839&dopt=Abstract

- **The use of aromatherapy in hospitalized children with HIV disease.**
  Author(s): Styles JL.
  Source: Complementary Therapies in Nursing & Midwifery. 1997 February; 3(1): 16-20. Review.
  http://www.ncbi.nlm.nih.gov:80/entrez/query.fcgi?cmd=Retrieve&db=PubMed&list_
  uids=9432422&dopt=Abstract

- **The use of aromatherapy in intrapartum midwifery practice an observational study.**
  Author(s): Burns E, Blamey C, Ersser SJ, Lloyd AJ, Barnetson L.
  Source: Complementary Therapies in Nursing & Midwifery. 2000 February; 6(1): 33-4.
  http://www.ncbi.nlm.nih.gov:80/entrez/query.fcgi?cmd=Retrieve&db=PubMed&list_
  uids=11033651&dopt=Abstract

- **The use of aromatherapy in wound care.**
  Author(s): Asquith S.
  Source: J Wound Care. 1999 June; 8(6): 318-20. Review. No Abstract Available.
  http://www.ncbi.nlm.nih.gov:80/entrez/query.fcgi?cmd=Retrieve&db=PubMed&list_
  uids=10776219&dopt=Abstract

- **Use of aromatherapy as a complementary treatment for chronic pain.**
  Author(s): Buckle J.
  Source: Alternative Therapies in Health and Medicine. 1999 September; 5(5): 42-51. Review.
  http://www.ncbi.nlm.nih.gov:80/entrez/query.fcgi?cmd=Retrieve&db=PubMed&list_
  uids=10484830&dopt=Abstract

- **Use of aromatherapy with hospice patients to decrease pain, anxiety, and depression and to promote an increased sense of well-being.**
  Author(s): Louis M, Kowalski SD.
  Source: Am J Hosp Palliat Care. 2002 November-December; 19(6): 381-6.
  http://www.ncbi.nlm.nih.gov:80/entrez/query.fcgi?cmd=Retrieve&db=PubMed&list_uids=12442972&dopt=Abstract

- **Using aromatherapy in the management of psoriasis.**
  Author(s): Walsh D.
  Source: Nursing Standard : Official Newspaper of the Royal College of Nursing. 1996 December 18; 11(13-15): 53-6.
  http://www.ncbi.nlm.nih.gov:80/entrez/query.fcgi?cmd=Retrieve&db=PubMed&list_uids=9000946&dopt=Abstract

- **Why aromatherapy works (even if it doesn't) and why we need less research.**
  Author(s): Vickers A.
  Source: The British Journal of General Practice : the Journal of the Royal College of General Practitioners. 2000 June; 50(455): 444-5.
  http://www.ncbi.nlm.nih.gov:80/entrez/query.fcgi?cmd=Retrieve&db=PubMed&list_uids=10962780&dopt=Abstract

- **Why aromatherapy works.**
  Author(s): Roberts L, Wilson S, Greenfield S.
  Source: The British Journal of General Practice : the Journal of the Royal College of General Practitioners. 2000 October; 50(459): 825-6.
  http://www.ncbi.nlm.nih.gov:80/entrez/query.fcgi?cmd=Retrieve&db=PubMed&list_uids=11127178&dopt=Abstract

- **Why aromatherapy works.**
  Author(s): Ernst E.
  Source: The British Journal of General Practice : the Journal of the Royal College of General Practitioners. 2000 October; 50(459): 825; Author Reply 826.
  http://www.ncbi.nlm.nih.gov:80/entrez/query.fcgi?cmd=Retrieve&db=PubMed&list_uids=11127177&dopt=Abstract

- **Will aromatherapy be a useful treatment strategy for people with multiple sclerosis who experience pain?**
  Author(s): Howarth AL.
  Source: Complementary Therapies in Nursing & Midwifery. 2002 August; 8(3): 138-41. Review.
  http://www.ncbi.nlm.nih.gov:80/entrez/query.fcgi?cmd=Retrieve&db=PubMed&list_uids=12353614&dopt=Abstract

- **Yes, but how do we know it's true? Knowledge claims in massage and aromatherapy.**
  Author(s): Vickers A.
  Source: Complementary Therapies in Nursing & Midwifery. 1997 June; 3(3): 63-5. Review.
  http://www.ncbi.nlm.nih.gov:80/entrez/query.fcgi?cmd=Retrieve&db=PubMed&list_uids=9439251&dopt=Abstract

CHAPTER 2. NUTRITION AND AROMATHERAPY

Overview

In this chapter, we will show you how to find studies dedicated specifically to nutrition and aromatherapy.

Finding Nutrition Studies on Aromatherapy

The National Institutes of Health's Office of Dietary Supplements (ODS) offers a searchable bibliographic database called the IBIDS (International Bibliographic Information on Dietary Supplements; National Institutes of Health, Building 31, Room 1B29, 31 Center Drive, MSC 2086, Bethesda, Maryland 20892-2086, Tel: 301-435-2920, Fax: 301-480-1845, E-mail: ods@nih.gov). The IBIDS contains over 460,000 scientific citations and summaries about dietary supplements and nutrition as well as references to published international, scientific literature on dietary supplements such as vitamins, minerals, and botanicals[4] The IBIDS includes references and citations to both human and animal research studies.

As a service of the ODS, access to the IBIDS database is available free of charge at the following Web address: **http://ods.od.nih.gov/databases/ibids.html** After entering the search area, you have three choices: (1) IBIDS Consumer Database, (2) Full IBIDS Database, or (3) Peer Reviewed Citations Only.

Now that you have selected a database, click on the "Advanced" tab. An advanced search allows you to retrieve up to 100 fully explained references in a comprehensive format. Type "aromatherapy" (or synonyms) into the search box, and click "Go." To narrow the search, you can also select the "Title" field.

---

[4] Adapted from **http://ods.od.nih.gov**. IBIDS is produced by the Office of Dietary Supplements (ODS) at the National Institutes of Health to assist the public, healthcare providers, educators, and researchers in locating credible, scientific information on dietary supplements. IBIDS was developed and will be maintained through an interagency partnership with the Food and Nutrition Information Center of the National Agricultural Library, U.S. Department of Agriculture.

The following information is typical of that found when using the "Full IBIDS Database" to search for "aromatherapy" (or a synonym):

- **A randomized trial of aromatherapy to reduce anxiety before abortion.**
  Author(s):   University   of   British   Columbia,   Vancouver,   Canada.
  ewiebe@interchange.ubc.ca
  Source: Wiebe, E Eff-Clin-Pract. 2000 Jul-August; 3(4): 166-9 1099-8128

- **A review of the literature surrounding the research into aromatherapy.**
  Author(s): Manchester College of Midwifery and Nursing.
  Source: Cawthorn, A Complement-Ther-Nurs-Midwifery. 1995 August; 1(4): 118-20 1353-6117

- **A study of the changes in the bioactivity of essential oils used singly and as mixtures in aromatherapy.**
  Author(s): School of Applied Science, South Bank University, London, UK.
  Source: Lis Balchin, M Deans, S Hart, S J-Altern-Complement-Med. 1997 Fall; 3(3): 249-56 1075-5535

- **Accidental bullous phototoxic reactions to bergamot aromatherapy oil.**
  Author(s): Department of Dermatology, University of Graz, Austria.
  Source: Kaddu, S Kerl, H Wolf, P J-Am-Acad-Dermatol. 2001 September; 45(3): 458-61 0190-9622

- **Allergic airborne contact dermatitis from essential oils used in aromatherapy.**
  Author(s): Dermatologic Clinic and Polyclinic of Ludwig-Maximilians-University, Munich, Germany.
  Source: Schaller, M Korting, H C Clin-Exp-Dermatol. 1995 March; 20(2): 143-5 0307-6938

- **Allergic contact dermatitis from aromatherapy.**
  Author(s): Department of Dermatology, Hospital of the University of Pennsylvania, Philadelphia, PA 19104, USA.
  Source: Weiss, R R James, W D Am-J-Contact-Dermat. 1997 December; 8(4): 250-1 1046-199X

- **An evaluation of aromatherapy massage in palliative care.**
  Author(s): Marie Curie Cancer Care, London, UK.
  Source: Wilkinson, S Aldridge, J Salmon, I Cain, E Wilson, B Palliat-Med. 1999 September; 13(5): 409-17 0269-2163

- **An investigation into the use of aromatherapy in intrapartum midwifery practice.**
  Author(s): Oxford Centre for Health Care Research and Development Oxford Brookes University, United Kingdom.
  Source: Burns, E E Blamey, C Ersser, S J Barnetson, L Lloyd, A J J-Altern-Complement-Med. 2000 April; 6(2): 141-7 1075-5535

- **Aromatherapy and its application in the management of people with dementia.**
  Source: Tobin, P Lampage 1995 June; 52(5): 34 0047-3936

- **Aromatherapy and massage.**
  Source: Hanse, M Nurs-Stand. 1990 August 22-28; 4(48): 43 0029-6570

- **Aromatherapy as a safe and effective treatment for the management of agitation in severe dementia: the results of a double-blind, placebo-controlled trial with Melissa.**
  Author(s): Wolfson Research Centre, Newcastle General Hospital, Institute for Ageing and Health, Newcastle upon Tyne, United Kingdom. c.g.ballard@ncl.ac.uk
  Source: Ballard, Clive G O'Brien, John T Reichelt, Katharina Perry, Elaine K J-Clin-Psychiatry. 2002 July; 63(7): 553-8 0160-6689

- **Aromatherapy for deaf and deafblind people living in residential accommodation.**
  Source: Armstrong, F Heidingsfeld, V Complement-Ther-Nurs-Midwifery. 2000 November; 6(4): 180-8 1353-6117

- **Aromatherapy for health professionals.**
  Source: Waterworth, S Aust-Nurs-J. 1999 September; 7(3): 37 1320-3185

- **Aromatherapy growing rapidly.**
  Source: Belcher, I Beginnings. 1996 February; 16(2): 4 1071-2984

- **Aromatherapy in midwifery: benefits and risks.**
  Author(s): University of Greenwich, Elizabeth Raybould Centre, Kent, UK.
  Source: Tiran, D Complement-Ther-Nurs-Midwifery. 1996 August; 2(4): 88-92 1353-6117

- **Aromatherapy in perianesthesia nursing.**
  Author(s): Oxford Brookes University, United Kingdom.
  Source: Buckle, J J-Perianesth-Nurs. 1999 December; 14(6): 336-44 1089-9472

- **Aromatherapy massage: its use in a ward setting.**
  Author(s): Acute Stroke Rehabilitation Unit, Guy's and St Thomas' Hospital NHS Trust, London.
  Source: Mullins, P Nurs-Times. 2002 May 28-June 3; 98(22): 36-7 0954-7762

- **Aromatherapy.**
  Source: Buckle, J Nurs-Times. 1993 May 19-25; 89(20): 32-5 0954-7762

- **Aromatherapy: the essentials (continuing education credit).**
  Source: Stevenson, C Nurs-Stand. 1994 November 23-29; 9(9 Suppl Nu): 3-8; quiz 11-3 0029-6570

- **Clinical aromatherapy and AIDS.**
  Author(s): RJ Buckle Associates LLC, Hunter, New York, USA.
  Source: Buckle, Jane J-Assoc-Nurses-AIDS-Care. 2002 May-June; 13(3): 81-99 1055-3290

- **Clinical aromatherapy and touch: complementary therapies for nursing practice.**
  Author(s): College of New Rochelle, New York, USA.
  Source: Buckle, J Crit-Care-Nurse. 1998 October; 18(5): 54-61 0279-5442

- **Clinical aromatherapy. Therapeutic uses for essential oils.**
  Author(s): RJ Buckle Associates, Catskills, N.Y., USA.
  Source: Buckle, J Adv-Nurse-Pract. 2002 May; 10(5): 67-8, 88 1096-6293

- **Complementary medicine. Aromatherapy.**
  Source: Trevelyan, J Booth, B Nurs-Times. 1994 September 21-27; 90(38): suppl 1-16 0954-7762

- **Complementary medicine. Using aromatherapy in childbirth.**
  Source: Burns, E Blamey, C Nurs-Times. 1994 March 2-8; 90(9): 54-60 0954-7762

- **Essential oils and 'aromatherapy': their modern role in healing.**
  Author(s): School of Applied Science, South Bank University, London.
  Source: Lis Balchin, M J-R-Soc-Health. 1997 October; 117(5): 324-9 0264-0325

- **Evaluation and attributional analysis of an aromatherapy service for older adults with physical health problems and carers using the service.**
  Author(s): South Birmingham Mental Health NHS Trust, UK.
  Source: Papadopoulos, A Wright, S Ensor, J Complement-Ther-Med. 1999 December; 7(4): 239-44 0965-2299

- **Holistic aromatherapy.**
  Source: Pounds, L Beginnings. 1992 March; 12(3): 1, 4 1071-2984

- **Measuring the effects of aromatherapy.**
  Source: Stevenson, C Nurs-Times. 1992 October 7-13; 88(41): 62-3 0954-7762

- **Possible health and safety problems in the use of novel plant essential oils and extracts in aromatherapy.**
  Author(s): South Bank University, London.
  Source: Lis Balchin, M J-R-Soc-Health. 1999 December; 119(4): 240-3 0264-0325

- **Prophylactic aromatherapy for supervening infections in patients with chronic bronchitis. Statistical evaluation conducted in clinics against a placebo.**
  Source: Ferley, J.P. Poutignat, N. Zmirou, D. Azzopardi, Y. Balducci, F. Phytother-Res-PTR. Sussex : John Wiley & Sons. June 1989. volume 3 (3) page 97-100. 0951-418X

- **Psychological effects of aromatherapy on chronic hemodialysis patients.**
  Author(s): Department of Neurophsyciatry, Hirosaki University Hospital, Japan.
  Source: Itai, T Amayasu, H Kuribayashi, M Kawamura, N Okada, M Momose, A Tateyama, T Narumi, K Uematsu, W Kaneko, S Psychiatry-Clin-Neurosci. 2000 August; 54(4): 393-7 1323-1316

- **Randomized trial of aromatherapy. Successful treatment for alopecia areata.**
  Author(s): Department of Dermatology, Aberdeen Royal Infirmary, Foresterhill, Scotland. ad.ormerod@abdn.ac.uk
  Source: Hay, I C Jamieson, M Ormerod, A D Arch-Dermatol. 1998 November; 134(11): 1349-52 0003-987X

- **Safe practice and aromatherapy.**
  Source: Maddocks, W Nurs-N-Z. 1995 November; 1(10): 15-6 1173-2032

- **Scientific status of aromatherapy.**
  Author(s): Department of Psychology, University of Warwick, Coventry, England.
  Source: King, J R Perspect-Biol-Med. 1994 Spring; 37(3): 409-15 0031-5982

- **Sensing an improvement: an experimental study to evaluate the use of aromatherapy, massage and periods of rest in an intensive care unit.**
  Author(s): Royal Bershire Hospital NHS Trust, Reading, England.
  Source: Dunn, C Sleep, J Collett, D J-Adv-Nurs. 1995 January; 21(1): 34-40 0309-2402

- **The development of clinical practice guidelines for the use of aromatherapy in a cancer setting.**
  Author(s): Peter MacCallum Cancer Institute, St Andrews Place, East Melbourne, VIC, 3002.
  Source: Campbell, L Pollard, A Roeton, C Aust-J-Holist-Nurs. 2001 April; 8(1): 14-22 1322-8803

- **The essence of aromatherapy.**
  Source: West, B Elder-Care. 1993 Jul-August; 5(4): 24-5 1369-1856

- **The role of aromatherapy in nursing care.**
  Author(s): Department of Botanical Medicine and Psychology, Bastyr University, Seattle, Washington. rjbinfo@aol.com
  Source: Buckle, J Nurs-Clin-North-Am. 2001 March; 36(1): 57-72 0029-6465

- **The science and art of aromatherapy.**
  Author(s): Virginia Commonwealth University/Medical College of Virginia Physicians, USA.
  Source: Robins, J L J-Holist-Nurs. 1999 March; 17(1): 5-17 0898-0101

- **The use of aromatherapy in hospitalized children with HIV disease.**
  Author(s): Paediatric Unit, St Mary's Hospital, London, UK.
  Source: Styles, J L Complement-Ther-Nurs-Midwifery. 1997 February; 3(1): 16-20 1353-6117

- **The use of aromatherapy in intrapartum midwifery practice an observational study.**
  Author(s): Oxford Brooks University, U.K.
  Source: Burns, E Blamey, C Ersser, S J Lloyd, A J Barnetson, L Complement-Ther-Nurs-Midwifery. 2000 February; 6(1): 33-4 1353-6117

- **Use of aromatherapy as a complementary treatment for chronic pain.**
  Source: Buckle, J Altern-Ther-Health-Med. 1999 September; 5(5): 42-51 1078-6791

- **Use of aromatherapy with hospice patients to decrease pain, anxiety, and depression and to promote an increased sense of well-being.**
  Author(s): Department of Nursing, University of Nevada, Las Vegas, USA.
  Source: Louis, M Kowalski, S D Am-J-Hosp-Palliat-Care. 2002 Nov-December; 19(6): 381-6 1049-9091

- **Using aromatherapy in the management of psoriasis.**
  Author(s): Homerton School of Health Studies, Cambridge.
  Source: Walsh, D Nurs-Stand. 1996 December 18; 11(13-15): 53-6 0029-6570

- **Will aromatherapy be a useful treatment strategy for people with multiple sclerosis who experience pain?**
  Author(s): Pain Management Service, Chelsea and Westminster Hospital, London, UK.
  amanda.howarth@chelwest.nhs.uk
  Source: Howarth, A L Complement-Ther-Nurs-Midwifery. 2002 August; 8(3): 138-41 1353-6117

Federal Resources on Nutrition

In addition to the IBIDS, the United States Department of Health and Human Services (HHS) and the United States Department of Agriculture (USDA) provide many sources of information on general nutrition and health. Recommended resources include:

- healthfinder®, HHS's gateway to health information, including diet and nutrition: **http://www.healthfinder.gov/scripts/SearchContext.asp?topic=238&page=0**

- The United States Department of Agriculture's Web site dedicated to nutrition information: **www.nutrition.gov**

- The Food and Drug Administration's Web site for federal food safety information: **www.foodsafety.gov**

- The National Action Plan on Overweight and Obesity sponsored by the United States Surgeon General: **http://www.surgeongeneral.gov/topics/obesity/**

- The Center for Food Safety and Applied Nutrition has an Internet site sponsored by the Food and Drug Administration and the Department of Health and Human Services: **http://vm.cfsan.fda.gov/**

- Center for Nutrition Policy and Promotion sponsored by the United States Department of Agriculture: **http://www.usda.gov/cnpp/**

- Food and Nutrition Information Center, National Agricultural Library sponsored by the United States Department of Agriculture: **http://www.nal.usda.gov/fnic/**

Food and Nutrition Service sponsored by the United States Department of Agriculture: **http://www.fns.usda.gov/fns/**

Additional Web Resources

A number of additional Web sites offer encyclopedic information covering food and nutrition. The following is a representative sample:

- AOL: **http://search.aol.com/cat.adp?id=174&layer=&from=subcats**
- Family Village: **http://www.familyvillage.wisc.edu/med_nutrition.html**
- Google: **http://directory.google.com/Top/Health/Nutrition/**
- Healthnotes: **http://www.healthnotes.com/**
- Open Directory Project: **http://dmoz.org/Health/Nutrition/**
- Yahoo.com: **http://dir.yahoo.com/Health/Nutrition/**
- WebMD®Health: **http://my.webmd.com/nutrition**
- WholeHealthMD.com: **http://www.wholehealthmd.com/reflib/0,1529,00.html**

CHAPTER 3. ALTERNATIVE MEDICINE AND AROMATHERAPY

Overview

In this chapter, we will begin by introducing you to official information sources on complementary and alternative medicine (CAM) relating to aromatherapy. At the conclusion of this chapter, we will provide additional sources.

The Combined Health Information Database

The Combined Health Information Database (CHID) is a bibliographic database produced by health-related agencies of the U.S. federal government (mostly from the National Institutes of Health) that can offer concise information for a targeted search. The CHID database is updated four times a year at the end of January, April, July, and October. Check the titles, summaries, and availability of CAM-related information by using the "Simple Search" option at the following Web site: **http://chid.nih.gov/simple/simple.html**. In the drop box at the top, select "Complementary and Alternative Medicine." Then type "aromatherapy" (or synonyms) in the second search box. We recommend that you select 100 "documents per page" and to check the "whole records" options. The following was extracted using this technique:

- **Complementary Therapies in Palliative Cancer Care**

  Source: Cancer. 91(11): 2181-2185. June 1, 2001.

  Summary: This journal article provides an overview of complementary therapies for palliative cancer care. First, it discusses the difference between alternative cancer 'cures' and complementary cancer care, including the potential dangers of alternative treatments and the goals of complementary medicine in palliative care. Then, it reviews evidence from exemplary studies and (where available) systematic reviews of selected complementary therapies used for palliative cancer care, including acupuncture, **aromatherapy,** enzyme therapy, homeopathy, hypnotherapy, massage, reflexology, relaxation, and spiritual healing. The author concludes that complementary medicine has some potential in palliative and supportive cancer care, although the evidence is not compelling for any of the therapies reviewed. He calls for further research in this area. The article has 1 table and 49 references.

National Center for Complementary and Alternative Medicine

The National Center for Complementary and Alternative Medicine (NCCAM) of the National Institutes of Health (http://nccam.nih.gov/) has created a link to the National Library of Medicine's databases to facilitate research for articles that specifically relate to aromatherapy and complementary medicine. To search the database, go to the following Web site: **http://www.nlm.nih.gov/nccam/camonpubmed.html.** Select "CAM on PubMed." Enter "aromatherapy" (or synonyms) into the search box. Click "Go." The following references provide information on particular aspects of complementary and alternative medicine that are related to aromatherapy:

- **A clinical trial of the effect of aromatherapy on motivational behaviour in a dementia care setting using a single subject design.**
  Author(s): MacMahon S, Kermode S.
  Source: Aust J Holist Nurs. 1998 October; 5(2): 47-9.
  http://www.ncbi.nlm.nih.gov:80/entrez/query.fcgi?cmd=Retrieve&db=PubMed&list_
  uids=10428895&dopt=Abstract

- **A pilot study addressing the effect of aromatherapy massage on mood, anxiety and relaxation in adult mental health.**
  Author(s): Edge J.
  Source: Complementary Therapies in Nursing & Midwifery. 2003 May; 9(2): 90-7.
  http://www.ncbi.nlm.nih.gov:80/entrez/query.fcgi?cmd=Retrieve&db=PubMed&list_
  uids=12697161&dopt=Abstract

- **A randomized trial of aromatherapy to reduce anxiety before abortion.**
  Author(s): Wiebe E.
  Source: Effective Clinical Practice : Ecp. 2000 July-August; 3(4): 166-9.
  http://www.ncbi.nlm.nih.gov:80/entrez/query.fcgi?cmd=Retrieve&db=PubMed&list_
  uids=11183431&dopt=Abstract

- **A review of the literature surrounding the research into aromatherapy.**
  Author(s): Cawthorn A.
  Source: Complementary Therapies in Nursing & Midwifery. 1995 August; 1(4): 118-20. Review.
  http://www.ncbi.nlm.nih.gov:80/entrez/query.fcgi?cmd=Retrieve&db=PubMed&list_
  uids=9456723&dopt=Abstract

- **A study of the changes in the bioactivity of essential oils used singly and as mixtures in aromatherapy.**
  Author(s): Lis-Balchin M, Deans S, Hart S.
  Source: Journal of Alternative and Complementary Medicine (New York, N.Y.). 1997 Fall; 3(3): 249-56.
  http://www.ncbi.nlm.nih.gov:80/entrez/query.fcgi?cmd=Retrieve&db=PubMed&list_
  uids=9430328&dopt=Abstract

- **Accidental bullous phototoxic reactions to bergamot aromatherapy oil.**
  Author(s): Kaddu S, Kerl H, Wolf P.
  Source: Journal of the American Academy of Dermatology. 2001 September; 45(3): 458-61.
  http://www.ncbi.nlm.nih.gov:80/entrez/query.fcgi?cmd=Retrieve&db=PubMed&list_uids=11511848&dopt=Abstract

- **Advancing my health care practice in aromatherapy.**
  Author(s): Clarke DA.
  Source: Aust J Holist Nurs. 1999 April; 6(1): 32-8.
  http://www.ncbi.nlm.nih.gov:80/entrez/query.fcgi?cmd=Retrieve&db=PubMed&list_uids=11898200&dopt=Abstract

- **Allergic airborne contact dermatitis from essential oils used in aromatherapy.**
  Author(s): Schaller M, Korting HC.
  Source: Clinical and Experimental Dermatology. 1995 March; 20(2): 143-5.
  http://www.ncbi.nlm.nih.gov:80/entrez/query.fcgi?cmd=Retrieve&db=PubMed&list_uids=8565250&dopt=Abstract

- **Allergic contact dermatitis from aromatherapy.**
  Author(s): Weiss RR, James WD.
  Source: American Journal of Contact Dermatitis : Official Journal of the American Contact Dermatitis Society. 1997 December; 8(4): 250-1.
  http://www.ncbi.nlm.nih.gov:80/entrez/query.fcgi?cmd=Retrieve&db=PubMed&list_uids=9358122&dopt=Abstract

- **An evaluation of aromatherapy massage in palliative care.**
  Author(s): Wilkinson S, Aldridge J, Salmon I, Cain E, Wilson B.
  Source: Palliative Medicine. 1999 September; 13(5): 409-17.
  http://www.ncbi.nlm.nih.gov:80/entrez/query.fcgi?cmd=Retrieve&db=PubMed&list_uids=10659113&dopt=Abstract

- **An investigation into the use of aromatherapy in intrapartum midwifery practice.**
  Author(s): Burns EE, Blamey C, Ersser SJ, Barnetson L, Lloyd AJ.
  Source: Journal of Alternative and Complementary Medicine (New York, N.Y.). 2000 April; 6(2): 141-7.
  http://www.ncbi.nlm.nih.gov:80/entrez/query.fcgi?cmd=Retrieve&db=PubMed&list_uids=10784271&dopt=Abstract

- **'Aroma 2000–fragrancing the future'. Favre Armstrong reports on the first Baltic States Aromatherapy Conference.**
  Author(s): Armstrong F.
  Source: Complementary Therapies in Nursing & Midwifery. 2001 May; 7(2): 104-7.
  http://www.ncbi.nlm.nih.gov:80/entrez/query.fcgi?cmd=Retrieve&db=PubMed&list_uids=11855769&dopt=Abstract

- **Aromatherapy again.**
  Author(s): Vickers A.

Source: The British Journal of General Practice : the Journal of the Royal College of General Practitioners. 2000 November; 50(460): 920.

http://www.ncbi.nlm.nih.gov:80/entrez/query.fcgi?cmd=Retrieve&db=PubMed&list_uids=11141888&dopt=Abstract

- **Aromatherapy and behaviour disturbances in dementia: a randomized controlled trial.**
  Author(s): Smallwood J, Brown R, Coulter F, Irvine E, Copland C.
  Source: International Journal of Geriatric Psychiatry. 2001 October; 16(10): 1010-3.
  http://www.ncbi.nlm.nih.gov:80/entrez/query.fcgi?cmd=Retrieve&db=PubMed&list_uids=11607948&dopt=Abstract

- **Aromatherapy and its application in cancer and palliative care.**
  Author(s): Cawthorn A, Carter A.
  Source: Complementary Therapies in Nursing & Midwifery. 2000 May; 6(2): 83-6.
  http://www.ncbi.nlm.nih.gov:80/entrez/query.fcgi?cmd=Retrieve&db=PubMed&list_uids=10844746&dopt=Abstract

- **Aromatherapy and its application in the management of people with dementia.**
  Author(s): Tobin P.
  Source: Lamp. 1995 June; 52(5): 34. No Abstract Available.
  http://www.ncbi.nlm.nih.gov:80/entrez/query.fcgi?cmd=Retrieve&db=PubMed&list_uids=7500733&dopt=Abstract

- **Aromatherapy and massage.**
  Author(s): Hanse M.
  Source: Nursing Standard : Official Newspaper of the Royal College of Nursing. 1990 August 22-28; 4(48): 43.
  http://www.ncbi.nlm.nih.gov:80/entrez/query.fcgi?cmd=Retrieve&db=PubMed&list_uids=2169854&dopt=Abstract

- **Aromatherapy and massage: the evidence.**
  Author(s): Buckle S.
  Source: Paediatric Nursing. 2003 July; 15(6): 24-7. Review.
  http://www.ncbi.nlm.nih.gov:80/entrez/query.fcgi?cmd=Retrieve&db=PubMed&list_uids=12889317&dopt=Abstract

- **Aromatherapy and the use of scents in psychotherapy.**
  Author(s): La Torre MA.
  Source: Perspectives in Psychiatric Care. 2003 January-March; 39(1): 35-7.
  http://www.ncbi.nlm.nih.gov:80/entrez/query.fcgi?cmd=Retrieve&db=PubMed&list_uids=12724965&dopt=Abstract

- **Aromatherapy as a safe and effective treatment for the management of agitation in severe dementia: the results of a double-blind, placebo-controlled trial with Melissa.**
  Author(s): Ballard CG, O'Brien JT, Reichelt K, Perry EK.
  Source: The Journal of Clinical Psychiatry. 2002 July; 63(7): 553-8.
  http://www.ncbi.nlm.nih.gov:80/entrez/query.fcgi?cmd=Retrieve&db=PubMed&list_uids=12143909&dopt=Abstract

- **Aromatherapy as an adjunct to care in a mental health day hospital.**
  Author(s): Hicks G.
  Source: Journal of Psychiatric and Mental Health Nursing. 1998 August; 5(4): 317.
  http://www.ncbi.nlm.nih.gov:80/entrez/query.fcgi?cmd=Retrieve&db=PubMed&list_uids=9807369&dopt=Abstract

- **Aromatherapy for deaf and deafblind people living in residential accommodation.**
  Author(s): Armstrong F, Heidingsfeld V.
  Source: Complementary Therapies in Nursing & Midwifery. 2000 November; 6(4): 180-8.
  http://www.ncbi.nlm.nih.gov:80/entrez/query.fcgi?cmd=Retrieve&db=PubMed&list_uids=11858301&dopt=Abstract

- **Aromatherapy for Health Professionals annual report.**
  Author(s): Buckle J.
  Source: Beginnings. 2001 January-February; 21(1): 9, 12. No Abstract Available.
  http://www.ncbi.nlm.nih.gov:80/entrez/query.fcgi?cmd=Retrieve&db=PubMed&list_uids=11898298&dopt=Abstract

- **Aromatherapy for health professionals.**
  Author(s): Buckle J.
  Source: Beginnings. 2003 January-February; 23(1): 6-7. No Abstract Available.
  http://www.ncbi.nlm.nih.gov:80/entrez/query.fcgi?cmd=Retrieve&db=PubMed&list_uids=12592972&dopt=Abstract

- **Aromatherapy for health professionals.**
  Author(s): Waterworth S.
  Source: Australian Nursing Journal (July 1993). 1999 September; 7(3): 37.
  http://www.ncbi.nlm.nih.gov:80/entrez/query.fcgi?cmd=Retrieve&db=PubMed&list_uids=11894265&dopt=Abstract

- **Aromatherapy for health professionals.**
  Author(s): Buckle J.
  Source: Beginnings. 2002 January-February; 22(1): 7. No Abstract Available.
  http://www.ncbi.nlm.nih.gov:80/entrez/query.fcgi?cmd=Retrieve&db=PubMed&list_uids=11842643&dopt=Abstract

- **Aromatherapy growing rapidly.**
  Author(s): Belcher I.
  Source: Beginnings. 1996 February; 16(2): 4. No Abstract Available.
  http://www.ncbi.nlm.nih.gov:80/entrez/query.fcgi?cmd=Retrieve&db=PubMed&list_uids=8704372&dopt=Abstract

- **Aromatherapy in arthritis: a study.**
  Author(s): Brownfield A.
  Source: Nursing Standard : Official Newspaper of the Royal College of Nursing. 1998 October 21-27; 13(5): 34-5.
  http://www.ncbi.nlm.nih.gov:80/entrez/query.fcgi?cmd=Retrieve&db=PubMed&list_uids=9919184&dopt=Abstract

- **Aromatherapy in dermatology.**
  Author(s): Stevensen CJ.
  Source: Clinics in Dermatology. 1998 November-December; 16(6): 689-94. Review.
  http://www.ncbi.nlm.nih.gov:80/entrez/query.fcgi?cmd=Retrieve&db=PubMed&list_
  uids=9949913&dopt=Abstract

- **Aromatherapy in midwifery: benefits and risks.**
  Author(s): Tiran D.
  Source: Complementary Therapies in Nursing & Midwifery. 1996 August; 2(4): 88-92.
  Review.
  http://www.ncbi.nlm.nih.gov:80/entrez/query.fcgi?cmd=Retrieve&db=PubMed&list_
  uids=9439282&dopt=Abstract

- **Aromatherapy in perianesthesia nursing.**
  Author(s): Buckle J.
  Source: Journal of Perianesthesia Nursing : Official Journal of the American Society of
  Perianesthesia Nurses / American Society of Perianesthesia Nurses. 1999 December;
  14(6): 336-44. Review.
  http://www.ncbi.nlm.nih.gov:80/entrez/query.fcgi?cmd=Retrieve&db=PubMed&list_
  uids=10839071&dopt=Abstract

- **Aromatherapy in practice.**
  Author(s): Avis A.
  Source: Nursing Standard : Official Newspaper of the Royal College of Nursing. 1999
  March 3-9; 13(24): 14-5.
  http://www.ncbi.nlm.nih.gov:80/entrez/query.fcgi?cmd=Retrieve&db=PubMed&list_
  uids=10335230&dopt=Abstract

- **Aromatherapy in practice: creative nursing care--Daw House Hospice.**
  Author(s): Osborne R.
  Source: Aust J Holist Nurs. 1998 October; 5(2): 50. No Abstract Available.
  http://www.ncbi.nlm.nih.gov:80/entrez/query.fcgi?cmd=Retrieve&db=PubMed&list_
  uids=10428896&dopt=Abstract

- **Aromatherapy in the care of older people.**
  Author(s): Brett H.
  Source: Nurs Times. 1999 August 18-24; 95(33): 56-7. No Abstract Available.
  http://www.ncbi.nlm.nih.gov:80/entrez/query.fcgi?cmd=Retrieve&db=PubMed&list_
  uids=10614423&dopt=Abstract

- **Aromatherapy massage for joint pain and constipation in a patient with Guillian
  Barre.**
  Author(s): Shirreffs CM.
  Source: Complementary Therapies in Nursing & Midwifery. 2001 May; 7(2): 78-83.
  http://www.ncbi.nlm.nih.gov:80/entrez/query.fcgi?cmd=Retrieve&db=PubMed&list_
  uids=11855776&dopt=Abstract

- **Aromatherapy massage: its use in a ward setting.**
  Author(s): Mullins P.

Source: Nurs Times. 2002 May 28-June 3; 98(22): 36-7. Review.
http://www.ncbi.nlm.nih.gov:80/entrez/query.fcgi?cmd=Retrieve&db=PubMed&list_
uids=12168454&dopt=Abstract

- **Aromatherapy positively affects mood, EEG patterns of alertness and math computations.**
  Author(s): Diego MA, Jones NA, Field T, Hernandez-Reif M, Schanberg S, Kuhn C, McAdam V, Galamaga R, Galamaga M.
  Source: The International Journal of Neuroscience. 1998 December; 96(3-4): 217-24.
  http://www.ncbi.nlm.nih.gov:80/entrez/query.fcgi?cmd=Retrieve&db=PubMed&list_
  uids=10069621&dopt=Abstract

- **Aromatherapy throughout history.**
  Author(s): El-Gammal SY.
  Source: Hamdard Med. 1990 April-June; 33(2): 41-61. No Abstract Available.
  http://www.ncbi.nlm.nih.gov:80/entrez/query.fcgi?cmd=Retrieve&db=PubMed&list_
  uids=11614003&dopt=Abstract

- **Aromatherapy.**
  Author(s): Eliopoulos C.
  Source: Director. 1999 Autumn; 7(4): 132. No Abstract Available.
  http://www.ncbi.nlm.nih.gov:80/entrez/query.fcgi?cmd=Retrieve&db=PubMed&list_
  uids=10703342&dopt=Abstract

- **Aromatherapy.**
  Author(s): Trevelyan J.
  Source: Nurs Times. 1993 June 23-29; 89(25): 38-40. No Abstract Available.
  http://www.ncbi.nlm.nih.gov:80/entrez/query.fcgi?cmd=Retrieve&db=PubMed&list_
  uids=8321693&dopt=Abstract

- **Aromatherapy.**
  Author(s): Buckle J.
  Source: Nurs Times. 1993 May 19-25; 89(20): 32-5.
  http://www.ncbi.nlm.nih.gov:80/entrez/query.fcgi?cmd=Retrieve&db=PubMed&list_
  uids=8321672&dopt=Abstract

- **Aromatherapy.**
  Author(s): Armstrong F.
  Source: Prof Nurse. 1986 August; 1(11): 305. No Abstract Available.
  http://www.ncbi.nlm.nih.gov:80/entrez/query.fcgi?cmd=Retrieve&db=PubMed&list_
  uids=3638730&dopt=Abstract

- **Aromatherapy. Introduction into a maternity service.**
  Author(s): Jardine M.
  Source: Pract Midwife. 2002 April; 5(4): 14-5. No Abstract Available.
  http://www.ncbi.nlm.nih.gov:80/entrez/query.fcgi?cmd=Retrieve&db=PubMed&list_
  uids=11987879&dopt=Abstract

- **Aromatherapy. Working with clients who are HIV positive.**
  Author(s): Toomer S.

Source: Nursing Standard : Official Newspaper of the Royal College of Nursing. 1994 April 20-26; 8(30): 83.
http://www.ncbi.nlm.nih.gov:80/entrez/query.fcgi?cmd=Retrieve&db=PubMed&list_uids=8003428&dopt=Abstract

- **Aromatherapy: a matter for debate.**
  Author(s): Hobbs S.
  Source: Complementary Therapies in Nursing & Midwifery. 1997 December; 3(6): 171.
  http://www.ncbi.nlm.nih.gov:80/entrez/query.fcgi?cmd=Retrieve&db=PubMed&list_uids=9511648&dopt=Abstract

- **Aromatherapy: a survey of current practice in the management of rheumatic disease symptoms.**
  Author(s): Osborn CE, Barlas P, Baxter GD, Barlow JH.
  Source: Complementary Therapies in Medicine. 2001 June; 9(2): 62-7.
  http://www.ncbi.nlm.nih.gov:80/entrez/query.fcgi?cmd=Retrieve&db=PubMed&list_uids=11444884&dopt=Abstract

- **Aromatherapy: a systematic review.**
  Author(s): Cooke B, Ernst E.
  Source: The British Journal of General Practice : the Journal of the Royal College of General Practitioners. 2000 June; 50(455): 493-6. Review.
  http://www.ncbi.nlm.nih.gov:80/entrez/query.fcgi?cmd=Retrieve&db=PubMed&list_uids=10962794&dopt=Abstract

- **Aromatherapy: evidence for sedative effects of the essential oil of lavender after inhalation.**
  Author(s): Buchbauer G, Jirovetz L, Jager W, Dietrich H, Plank C.
  Source: Z Naturforsch [c]. 1991 November-December; 46(11-12): 1067-72.
  http://www.ncbi.nlm.nih.gov:80/entrez/query.fcgi?cmd=Retrieve&db=PubMed&list_uids=1817516&dopt=Abstract

- **Aromatherapy: ineffective treatment or effective placebo?**
  Author(s): Bent S.
  Source: Effective Clinical Practice : Ecp. 2000 July-August; 3(4): 188-90.
  http://www.ncbi.nlm.nih.gov:80/entrez/query.fcgi?cmd=Retrieve&db=PubMed&list_uids=11183435&dopt=Abstract

- **Aromatherapy: is it for real?**
  Author(s): Cerrato PL.
  Source: Rn. 1998 June; 61(6): 51-2. Review.
  http://www.ncbi.nlm.nih.gov:80/entrez/query.fcgi?cmd=Retrieve&db=PubMed&list_uids=9668906&dopt=Abstract

- **Aromatherapy: mythical, magical, or medicinal?**
  Author(s): Thomas DV.
  Source: Holistic Nursing Practice. 2002 October; 16(5): 8-16. Review.
  http://www.ncbi.nlm.nih.gov:80/entrez/query.fcgi?cmd=Retrieve&db=PubMed&list_uids=12465213&dopt=Abstract

- **Aromatherapy: the essentials (continuing education credit).**
  Author(s): Stevenson C.
  Source: Nursing Standard : Official Newspaper of the Royal College of Nursing. 1994 November 23-29; 9(9 Suppl Nu): 3-8; Quiz 11-3.
  http://www.ncbi.nlm.nih.gov:80/entrez/query.fcgi?cmd=Retrieve&db=PubMed&list_uids=7811632&dopt=Abstract

- **Aromatherapy: the scents for survival.**
  Author(s): Buckle J.
  Source: Beginnings. 1994 May; 14(5): 1, 7. No Abstract Available.
  http://www.ncbi.nlm.nih.gov:80/entrez/query.fcgi?cmd=Retrieve&db=PubMed&list_uids=7795337&dopt=Abstract

- **Aromatherapy: the smell of success. Interview by Jackie O'Byrne.**
  Author(s): Clifford F.
  Source: Nursing Standard : Official Newspaper of the Royal College of Nursing. 1990 August 15-21; 4(47): 23.
  http://www.ncbi.nlm.nih.gov:80/entrez/query.fcgi?cmd=Retrieve&db=PubMed&list_uids=2169853&dopt=Abstract

- **Aromatherapy: therapeutic applications of plant essential oils.**
  Author(s): Halcon LL.
  Source: Minn Med. 2002 November; 85(11): 42-6.
  http://www.ncbi.nlm.nih.gov:80/entrez/query.fcgi?cmd=Retrieve&db=PubMed&list_uids=12498066&dopt=Abstract

- **Aromatherapy--nice but not 'essential'.**
  Author(s): Mackereth P.
  Source: Complementary Therapies in Nursing & Midwifery. 1995 February; 1(1): 47. Review.
  http://www.ncbi.nlm.nih.gov:80/entrez/query fcgi?cmd=Retrieve&db=PubMed&list_uids=9456699&dopt=Abstract

- **Can aromatherapy replace pre-medication?**
  Author(s): Gibbons E.
  Source: Br J Theatre Nurs. 1998 August; 8(5): 34-6. Review.
  http://www.ncbi.nlm.nih.gov:80/entrez/query.fcgi?cmd=Retrieve&db=PubMed&list_uids=9782829&dopt=Abstract

- **Cancer patients' experiences and evaluations of aromatherapy massage in palliative care.**
  Author(s): Dunwoody L, Smyth A, Davidson R.
  Source: International Journal of Palliative Nursing. 2002 October; 8(10): 497-504.
  http://www.ncbi.nlm.nih.gov:80/entrez/query.fcgi?cmd=Retrieve&db=PubMed&list_uids=12419989&dopt=Abstract

- **Clinical aromatherapy and AIDS.**
  Author(s): Buckle J.

Source: The Journal of the Association of Nurses in Aids Care : Janac. 2002 May-June; 13(3): 81-99.
http://www.ncbi.nlm.nih.gov:80/entrez/query.fcgi?cmd=Retrieve&db=PubMed&list_uids=12064023&dopt=Abstract

- **Clinical aromatherapy and touch: complementary therapies for nursing practice.**
Author(s): Buckle J.
Source: Critical Care Nurse. 1998 October; 18(5): 54-61. Review.
http://www.ncbi.nlm.nih.gov:80/entrez/query.fcgi?cmd=Retrieve&db=PubMed&list_uids=9934050&dopt=Abstract

- **Clinical aromatherapy. Therapeutic uses for essential oils.**
Author(s): Buckle J.
Source: Adv Nurse Pract. 2002 May; 10(5): 67-8, 88. Review. No Abstract Available.
http://www.ncbi.nlm.nih.gov:80/entrez/query.fcgi?cmd=Retrieve&db=PubMed&list_uids=12420533&dopt=Abstract

- **Complementary medicine. Aromatherapy.**
Author(s): Trevelyan J, Booth B.
Source: Nurs Times. 1994 September 21-27; 90(38): Suppl 1-16. No Abstract Available.
http://www.ncbi.nlm.nih.gov:80/entrez/query.fcgi?cmd=Retrieve&db=PubMed&list_uids=7971321&dopt=Abstract

- **Complementary medicine. Using aromatherapy in childbirth.**
Author(s): Burns E, Blamey C.
Source: Nurs Times. 1994 March 2-8; 90(9): 54-60. No Abstract Available.
http://www.ncbi.nlm.nih.gov:80/entrez/query.fcgi?cmd=Retrieve&db=PubMed&list_uids=8152975&dopt=Abstract

- **Complementary therapies in nursing. Implications for practice using aromatherapy as an example.**
Author(s): Johnson GR.
Source: Complementary Therapies in Nursing & Midwifery. 1995 October; 1(5): 128-32. Review.
http://www.ncbi.nlm.nih.gov:80/entrez/query.fcgi?cmd=Retrieve&db=PubMed&list_uids=9456726&dopt=Abstract

- **Complementary therapy: aromatherapy with massage for geriatric and hospice care--a call for an holistic approach.**
Author(s): Howdyshell C.
Source: Hosp J. 1998; 13(3): 69-75. Review.
http://www.ncbi.nlm.nih.gov:80/entrez/query.fcgi?cmd=Retrieve&db=PubMed&list_uids=9677958&dopt=Abstract

- **Contemporary therapy: aromatherapy in the management of acute pain?**
Author(s): Ching M.
Source: Contemp Nurse. 1999 December; 8(4): 146-51.
http://www.ncbi.nlm.nih.gov:80/entrez/query.fcgi?cmd=Retrieve&db=PubMed&list_uids=11141786&dopt=Abstract

- **Development of an aromatherapy service at a Cancer Centre.**
  Author(s): Kite SM, Maher EJ, Anderson K, Young T, Young J, Wood J, Howells N, Bradburn J.
  Source: Palliative Medicine. 1998 May; 12(3): 171-80.
  http://www.ncbi.nlm.nih.gov:80/entrez/query.fcgi?cmd=Retrieve&db=PubMed&list_uids=9743836&dopt=Abstract

- **Down to basics: the question of base gels and creams for aromatherapy. Interview by Caroline Stevensen.**
  Author(s): Kusmirek J.
  Source: Complementary Therapies in Nursing & Midwifery. 1998 August; 4(4): 118-9.
  http://www.ncbi.nlm.nih.gov:80/entrez/query.fcgi?cmd=Retrieve&db=PubMed&list_uids=9830939&dopt=Abstract

- **Enhancing care using aromatherapy.**
  Author(s): Spurling S.
  Source: Br J Theatre Nurs. 1998 July; 8(4): 36-8. Review. No Abstract Available.
  http://www.ncbi.nlm.nih.gov:80/entrez/query.fcgi?cmd=Retrieve&db=PubMed&list_uids=9782820&dopt=Abstract

- **Essential oils and 'aromatherapy': their modern role in healing.**
  Author(s): Lis-Balchin M.
  Source: J R Soc Health. 1997 October; 117(5): 324-9. Review.
  http://www.ncbi.nlm.nih.gov:80/entrez/query.fcgi?cmd=Retrieve&db=PubMed&list_uids=9519666&dopt=Abstract

- **Evaluation and attributional analysis of an aromatherapy service for older adults with physical health problems and carers using the service.**
  Author(s): Papadopoulos A, Wright S, Ensor J.
  Source: Complementary Therapies in Medicine. 1999 December; 7(4): 239-44.
  http://www.ncbi.nlm.nih.gov:80/entrez/query.fcgi?cmd=Retrieve&db=PubMed&list_uids=10709309&dopt=Abstract

- **Experiences with aromatherapy in the elderly.**
  Author(s): O'Brien B.
  Source: Journal of Alternative and Complementary Medicine (New York, N.Y.). 1997 Fall; 3(3): 211.
  http://www.ncbi.nlm.nih.gov:80/entrez/query.fcgi?cmd=Retrieve&db=PubMed&list_uids=9430321&dopt=Abstract

- **Formation and development of the Aromatherapy Organisations Council.**
  Author(s): Baker S.
  Source: Complementary Therapies in Nursing & Midwifery. 1997 June; 3(3): 77-80.
  http://www.ncbi.nlm.nih.gov:80/entrez/query.fcgi?cmd=Retrieve&db=PubMed&list_uids=9439254&dopt=Abstract

- **Holistic aromatherapy.**
  Author(s): Pounds L.

Source: Beginnings. 1992 March; 12(3): 1, 4. No Abstract Available.
http://www.ncbi.nlm.nih.gov:80/entrez/query.fcgi?cmd=Retrieve&db=PubMed&list_
uids=1551007&dopt=Abstract

- **Implementing aromatherapy in nursing and midwifery practice.**
  Author(s): Rawlings F, Meerabeau L.
  Source: Journal of Clinical Nursing. 2003 May; 12(3): 405-11.
  http://www.ncbi.nlm.nih.gov:80/entrez/query.fcgi?cmd=Retrieve&db=PubMed&list_
  uids=12709115&dopt=Abstract

- **Influence of aromatherapy on medication administration to residential-care residents with dementia and behavioral challenges.**
  Author(s): Gray SG, Clair AA.
  Source: Am J Alzheimers Dis Other Demen. 2002 May-June; 17(3): 169-74.
  http://www.ncbi.nlm.nih.gov:80/entrez/query.fcgi?cmd=Retrieve&db=PubMed&list_
  uids=12083347&dopt=Abstract

- **Inhalation aromatherapy during radiotherapy: results of a placebo-controlled double-blind randomized trial.**
  Author(s): Graham PH, Browne L, Cox H, Graham J.
  Source: Journal of Clinical Oncology : Official Journal of the American Society of Clinical Oncology. 2003 June 15; 21(12): 2372-6.
  http://www.ncbi.nlm.nih.gov:80/entrez/query.fcgi?cmd=Retrieve&db=PubMed&list_
  uids=12805340&dopt=Abstract

- **Lavender aromatherapy in recovery from exercise.**
  Author(s): Romine IJ, Bush AM, Geist CR.
  Source: Percept Mot Skills. 1999 June; 88(3 Pt 1): 756-8.
  http://www.ncbi.nlm.nih.gov:80/entrez/query.fcgi?cmd=Retrieve&db=PubMed&list_
  uids=10407881&dopt=Abstract

- **Learning the hard way! Setting up an RCT of aromatherapy massage for patients with advanced cancer.**
  Author(s): Westcombe AM, Gambles MA, Wilkinson SM, Barnes K, Fellowes D, Maher EJ, Young T, Love SB, Lucey RA, Cubbin S, Ramirez AJ.
  Source: Palliative Medicine. 2003 June; 17(4): 300-7.
  http://www.ncbi.nlm.nih.gov:80/entrez/query.fcgi?cmd=Retrieve&db=PubMed&list_
  uids=12822844&dopt=Abstract

- **Massage and aromatherapy massage: nursing art and science.**
  Author(s): Buckley J.
  Source: International Journal of Palliative Nursing. 2002 June; 8(6): 276-80. Review.
  http://www.ncbi.nlm.nih.gov:80/entrez/query.fcgi?cmd=Retrieve&db=PubMed&list_
  uids=12131821&dopt=Abstract

- **Massage and aromatherapy on a leukaemia unit.**
  Author(s): Stringer J.

Source: Complementary Therapies in Nursing & Midwifery. 2000 May; 6(2): 72-6.
http://www.ncbi.nlm.nih.gov:80/entrez/query.fcgi?cmd=Retrieve&db=PubMed&list_
uids=10844744&dopt=Abstract

- **Measuring the effects of aromatherapy.**
  Author(s): Stevenson C.
  Source: Nurs Times. 1992 October 7-13; 88(41): 62-3. No Abstract Available.
  http://www.ncbi.nlm.nih.gov:80/entrez/query.fcgi?cmd=Retrieve&db=PubMed&list_
  uids=1491983&dopt=Abstract

- **Patients' views on the factors which would influence the use of an aromatherapy massage out-patient service.**
  Author(s): Kacperek L.
  Source: Complementary Therapies in Nursing & Midwifery. 1997 April; 3(2): 51-7.
  http://www.ncbi.nlm.nih.gov:80/entrez/query.fcgi?cmd=Retrieve&db=PubMed&list_
  uids=9432431&dopt=Abstract

- **Phototoxic contact dermatitis from 5-methoxypsoralen in aromatherapy oil.**
  Author(s): Clark SM, Wilkinson SM.
  Source: Contact Dermatitis. 1998 May; 38(5): 289-90.
  http://www.ncbi.nlm.nih.gov:80/entrez/query.fcgi?cmd=Retrieve&db=PubMed&list_
  uids=9667455&dopt=Abstract

- **Possible health and safety problems in the use of novel plant essential oils and extracts in aromatherapy.**
  Author(s): Lis-Balchin M.
  Source: J R Soc Health. 1999 December; 119(4): 240-3. Review.
  http://www.ncbi.nlm.nih.gov:80/entrez/query.fcgi?cmd=Retrieve&db=PubMed&list_
  uids=10673845&dopt=Abstract

- **Psychological effects of aromatherapy on chronic hemodialysis patients.**
  Author(s): Itai T, Amayasu H, Kuribayashi M, Kawamura N, Okada M, Momose A, Tateyama T, Narumi K, Uematsu W, Kaneko S.
  Source: Psychiatry and Clinical Neurosciences. 2000 August; 54(4): 393-7.
  http://www.ncbi.nlm.nih.gov:80/entrez/query.fcgi?cmd=Retrieve&db=PubMed&list_
  uids=10997854&dopt=Abstract

- **Randomized trial of aromatherapy. Successful treatment for alopecia areata.**
  Author(s): Hay IC, Jamieson M, Ormerod AD.
  Source: Archives of Dermatology. 1998 November; 134(11): 1349-52.
  http://www.ncbi.nlm.nih.gov:80/entrez/query.fcgi?cmd=Retrieve&db=PubMed&list_
  uids=9828867&dopt=Abstract

- **Randomized trial of aromatherapy: successful treatment for alopecia areata.**
  Author(s): Kalish RS.
  Source: Archives of Dermatology. 1999 May; 135(5): 602-3.
  http://www.ncbi.nlm.nih.gov:80/entrez/query.fcgi?cmd=Retrieve&db=PubMed&list_
  uids=10328210&dopt=Abstract

- **Re: Essential oils and 'aromatherapy' their modern role in healing.**
  Author(s): Lis-Balchin M.
  Source: J R Soc Health. 1998 April; 118(2): 126. No Abstract Available.
  http://www.ncbi.nlm.nih.gov:80/entrez/query.fcgi?cmd=Retrieve&db=PubMed&list_uids=10076647&dopt=Abstract

- **Re: Essential oils and 'aromatherapy': their role in healing.**
  Author(s): Packham CL.
  Source: J R Soc Health. 1997 December; 117(6): 400. No Abstract Available.
  http://www.ncbi.nlm.nih.gov:80/entrez/query.fcgi?cmd=Retrieve&db=PubMed&list_uids=9519679&dopt=Abstract

- **Safe practice and aromatherapy.**
  Author(s): Maddocks W.
  Source: Nurs N Z. 1995 November; 1(10): 15-6. No Abstract Available.
  http://www.ncbi.nlm.nih.gov:80/entrez/query.fcgi?cmd=Retrieve&db=PubMed&list_uids=8536097&dopt=Abstract

- **Scents or nonsense: aromatherapy's benefits still subject to debate.**
  Author(s): Nelson NJ.
  Source: Journal of the National Cancer Institute. 1997 September 17; 89(18): 1334-6.
  http://www.ncbi.nlm.nih.gov:80/entrez/query.fcgi?cmd=Retrieve&db=PubMed&list_uids=9308699&dopt=Abstract

- **Scientific status of aromatherapy.**
  Author(s): King JR.
  Source: Perspectives in Biology and Medicine. 1994 Spring; 37(3): 409-15.
  http://www.ncbi.nlm.nih.gov:80/entrez/query.fcgi?cmd=Retrieve&db=PubMed&list_uids=8202345&dopt=Abstract

- **Sensing an improvement: an experimental study to evaluate the use of aromatherapy, massage and periods of rest in an intensive care unit.**
  Author(s): Dunn C, Sleep J, Collett D.
  Source: Journal of Advanced Nursing. 1995 January; 21(1): 34-40.
  http://www.ncbi.nlm.nih.gov:80/entrez/query.fcgi?cmd=Retrieve&db=PubMed&list_uids=7897075&dopt=Abstract

- **Should there be aromatherapy for addiction?**
  Author(s): Miller WR, Walker DD.
  Source: Addiction (Abingdon, England). 1997 April; 92(4): 486-7.
  http://www.ncbi.nlm.nih.gov:80/entrez/query.fcgi?cmd=Retrieve&db=PubMed&list_uids=9177073&dopt=Abstract

- **Single case evaluation of the effects of aromatherapy and massage on disturbed behaviour in severe dementia.**
  Author(s): Brooker DJ, Snape M, Johnson E, Ward D, Payne M.

Source: The British Journal of Clinical Psychology / the British Psychological Society. 1997 May; 36 (Pt 2): 287-96.
http://www.ncbi.nlm.nih.gov:80/entrez/query.fcgi?cmd=Retrieve&db=PubMed&list_uids=9167869&dopt=Abstract

- **The clinical use of aromatherapy in the reduction of stress.**
  Author(s): Rimmer L.
  Source: Home Healthcare Nurse. 1998 February; 16(2): 123-6.
  http://www.ncbi.nlm.nih.gov:80/entrez/query.fcgi?cmd=Retrieve&db=PubMed&list_uids=9526345&dopt=Abstract

- **The development of clinical practice guidelines for the use of aromatherapy in a cancer setting.**
  Author(s): Campbell L, Pollard A, Roeton C.
  Source: Aust J Holist Nurs. 2001 April; 8(1): 14-22. Review.
  http://www.ncbi.nlm.nih.gov:80/entrez/query.fcgi?cmd=Retrieve&db=PubMed&list_uids=11898289&dopt=Abstract

- **The effect of aromatherapy in promoting relaxation and stress reduction in a general hospital.**
  Author(s): Cannard G.
  Source: Complementary Therapies in Nursing & Midwifery. 1996 April; 2(2): 38-40.
  http://www.ncbi.nlm.nih.gov:80/entrez/query fcgi?cmd=Retrieve&db=PubMed&list_uids=9439271&dopt=Abstract

- **The effects of aromatherapy on pruritus in patients undergoing hemodialysis.**
  Author(s): Ro YJ, Ha HC, Kim CG, Yeom HA.
  Source: Dermatology Nursing / Dermatology Nurses' Association. 2002 August; 14(4): 231-4, 237-8, 256; Quiz 239.
  http://www.ncbi.nlm.nih.gov:80/entrez/query.fcgi?cmd=Retrieve&db=PubMed&list_uids=12240499&dopt=Abstract

- **The essence of aromatherapy.**
  Author(s): West B.
  Source: Elder Care. 1993 July-August; 5(4): 24-5. No Abstract Available.
  http://www.ncbi.nlm.nih.gov:80/entrez/query.fcgi?cmd=Retrieve&db=PubMed&list_uids=8348128&dopt=Abstract

- **The promise of aromatherapy. Essential oils have been shown in clinical trials to soothe some chronic ills brought on by old age.**
  Author(s): Wood K.
  Source: Provider. 2003 March; 29(3): 47-8. No Abstract Available.
  http://www.ncbi.nlm.nih.gov:80/entrez/query.fcgi?cmd=Retrieve&db=PubMed&list_uids=12666332&dopt=Abstract

- **The role of aromatherapy in nursing care.**
  Author(s): Buckle J.

Source: Nurs Clin North Am. 2001 March; 36(1): 57-72. Review.
http://www.ncbi.nlm.nih.gov:80/entrez/query.fcgi?cmd=Retrieve&db=PubMed&list_
uids=11342402&dopt=Abstract

- **The role of aromatherapy massage in reducing anxiety in patients with malignant brain tumours.**
  Author(s): Hadfield N.
  Source: International Journal of Palliative Nursing. 2001 June; 7(6): 279-85. Review.
  http://www.ncbi.nlm.nih.gov:80/entrez/query.fcgi?cmd=Retrieve&db=PubMed&list_
  uids=12066022&dopt=Abstract

- **The science and art of aromatherapy.**
  Author(s): Robins JL.
  Source: Journal of Holistic Nursing : Official Journal of the American Holistic Nurses' Association. 1999 March; 17(1): 5-17. Review.
  http://www.ncbi.nlm.nih.gov:80/entrez/query.fcgi?cmd=Retrieve&db=PubMed&list_
  uids=10373839&dopt=Abstract

- **The use of aromatherapy in hospitalized children with HIV disease.**
  Author(s): Styles JL.
  Source: Complementary Therapies in Nursing & Midwifery. 1997 February; 3(1): 16-20. Review.
  http://www.ncbi.nlm.nih.gov:80/entrez/query.fcgi?cmd=Retrieve&db=PubMed&list_
  uids=9432422&dopt=Abstract

- **The use of aromatherapy in intrapartum midwifery practice an observational study.**
  Author(s): Burns E, Blamey C, Ersser SJ, Lloyd AJ, Barnetson L.
  Source: Complementary Therapies in Nursing & Midwifery. 2000 February; 6(1): 33-4.
  http://www.ncbi.nlm.nih.gov:80/entrez/query.fcgi?cmd=Retrieve&db=PubMed&list_
  uids=11033651&dopt=Abstract

- **The use of aromatherapy in wound care.**
  Author(s): Asquith S.
  Source: J Wound Care. 1999 June; 8(6): 318-20. Review. No Abstract Available.
  http://www.ncbi.nlm.nih.gov:80/entrez/query.fcgi?cmd=Retrieve&db=PubMed&list_
  uids=10776219&dopt=Abstract

- **Use of aromatherapy as a complementary treatment for chronic pain.**
  Author(s): Buckle J.
  Source: Alternative Therapies in Health and Medicine. 1999 September; 5(5): 42-51. Review.
  http://www.ncbi.nlm.nih.gov:80/entrez/query.fcgi?cmd=Retrieve&db=PubMed&list_
  uids=10484830&dopt=Abstract

- **Use of aromatherapy with hospice patients to decrease pain, anxiety, and depression and to promote an increased sense of well-being.**
  Author(s): Louis M, Kowalski SD.

Source: Am J Hosp Palliat Care. 2002 November-December; 19(6): 381-6.
http://www.ncbi.nlm.nih.gov:80/entrez/query.fcgi?cmd=Retrieve&db=PubMed&list_
uids=12442972&dopt=Abstract

 Using aromatherapy in the management of psoriasis.
Author(s): Walsh D.
Source: Nursing Standard : Official Newspaper of the Royal College of Nursing. 1996
December 18; 11(13-15): 53-6.
http://www.ncbi.nlm.nih.gov:80/entrez/query.fcgi?cmd=Retrieve&db=PubMed&list_
uids=9000946&dopt=Abstract

- **Why aromatherapy works (even if it doesn't) and why we need less research.**
  Author(s): Vickers A.
  Source: The British Journal of General Practice : the Journal of the Royal College of
  General Practitioners. 2000 June; 50(455): 444-5.
  http://www.ncbi.nlm.nih.gov:80/entrez/query.fcgi?cmd=Retrieve&db=PubMed&list_
  uids=10962780&dopt=Abstract

- **Why aromatherapy works.**
  Author(s): Roberts L, Wilson S, Greenfield S.
  Source: The British Journal of General Practice : the Journal of the Royal College of
  General Practitioners. 2000 October; 50(459): 825-6.
  http://www.ncbi.nlm.nih.gov:80/entrez/query.fcgi?cmd=Retrieve&db=PubMed&list_
  uids=11127178&dopt=Abstract

- **Why aromatherapy works.**
  Author(s): Ernst E.
  Source: The British Journal of General Practice : the Journal of the Royal College of
  General Practitioners. 2000 October; 50(459): 825; Author Reply 826.
  http://www.ncbi.nlm.nih.gov:80/entrez/query.fcgi?cmd=Retrieve&db=PubMed&list_
  uids=11127177&dopt=Abstract

- **Will aromatherapy be a useful treatment strategy for people with multiple sclerosis
  who experience pain?**
  Author(s): Howarth AL.
  Source: Complementary Therapies in Nursing & Midwifery. 2002 August; 8(3): 138-41.
  Review.
  http://www.ncbi.nlm.nih.gov:80/entrez/query.fcgi?cmd=Retrieve&db=PubMed&list_
  uids=12353614&dopt=Abstract

- **Yes, but how do we know it's true? Knowledge claims in massage and aromatherapy.**
  Author(s): Vickers A.
  Source: Complementary Therapies in Nursing & Midwifery. 1997 June; 3(3): 63-5.

Additional Web Resources

A number of additional Web sites offer encyclopedic information covering CAM and related topics. The following is a representative sample:

- Alternative Medicine Foundation, Inc.: **http://www.herbmed.org/**

- AOL: **http://search.aol.com/cat.adp?id=169&layer=&from=subcats**

- Chinese Medicine: **http://www.newcenturynutrition.com/**

- drkoop.com®: **http://www.drkoop.com/InteractiveMedicine/IndexC.html**

- Family Village: **http://www.familyvillage.wisc.edu/med_altn.htm**

- Google: **http://directory.google.com/Top/Health/Alternative/**

- Healthnotes: **http://www.healthnotes.com/**

- MedWebPlus:
  http://medwebplus.com/subject/Alternative_and_Complementary_Medicine

- Open Directory Project: **http://dmoz.org/Health/Alternative/**

- HealthGate: **http://www.tnp.com/**

- WebMD®Health: **http://my.webmd.com/drugs_and_herbs**

- WholeHealthMD.com: **http://www.wholehealthmd.com/reflib/0,1529,00.html**

- Yahoo.com: **http://dir.yahoo.com/Health/Alternative_Medicine/**

The following is a specific Web list relating to aromatherapy; please note that any particular subject below may indicate either a therapeutic use, or a contraindication (potential danger), and does not reflect an official recommendation:

- **General Overview**

  Alopecia
  Source: Integrative Medicine Communications; www.drkoop.com

  Anxiety
  Source: Integrative Medicine Communications; www.drkoop.com

  Brain Cancer
  Source: Integrative Medicine Communications; www.drkoop.com

  Bronchitis
  Source: Healthnotes, Inc. www.healthnotes.com

  Cancer, Brain
  Source: Integrative Medicine Communications; www.drkoop.com

  Chronic Fatigue Syndrome
  Source: Integrative Medicine Communications; www.drkoop.com

Depression
Source: Integrative Medicine Communications; www.drkoop.com

Fatigue, Chronic Syndrome
Source: Integrative Medicine Communications; www.drkoop.com

Fibromyalgia
Source: Integrative Medicine Communications; www.drkoop.com

Hair Disorders
Source: Integrative Medicine Communications; www.drkoop.com

Hair Loss
Source: Integrative Medicine Communications; www.drkoop.com

Insomnia
Source: Healthnotes, Inc. www.healthnotes.com

- **Alternative Therapy**

  30-Day Body Purification Program
  Source: The Canoe version of A Dictionary of Alternative-Medicine Methods, by
  Priorities for Health editor Jack Raso, M.S., R.D.
  Hyperlink: http://www.canoe.ca/AltmedDictionary/t.html

  Aroma Behavior Conditioning
  Alternative names: ABC
  Source: The Canoe version of A Dictionary of Alternative-Medicine Methods, by
  Priorities for Health editor Jack Raso, M.S., R.D.
  Hyperlink: http://www.canoe.ca/AltmedDictionary/a.html

  Aroma-Genera
  Alternative names: Aroma-Genera system
  Source: The Canoe version of A Dictionary of Alternative-Medicine Methods, by
  Priorities for Health editor Jack Raso, M.S., R.D.
  Hyperlink: http://www.canoe.ca/AltmedDictionary/a.html

  Aroma-spa therapy
  Source: The Canoe version of A Dictionary of Alternative-Medicine Methods, by
  Priorities for Health editor Jack Raso, M.S., R.D.
  Hyperlink: http://www.canoe.ca/AltmedDictionary/a.html

  Aromatherapy
  Source: Healthnotes, Inc. www.healthnotes.com

  Aromatherapy
  Source: Integrative Medicine Communications; www.drkoop.com

Aromatherapy
Alternative names: aromatic medicine conventional aromatherapy holistic aromatherapy
Source: The Canoe version of A Dictionary of Alternative-Medicine Methods, by Priorities for Health editor Jack Raso, M.S., R.D.
Hyperlink: http://www.canoe.ca/AltmedDictionary/a.html

Aromatherapy
Source: WholeHealthMD.com, LLC. www.wholehealthmd.com
Hyperlink:
http://www.wholehealthmd.com/refshelf/substances_view/0,1525,664,00.html

Aroma-tology
Source: The Canoe version of A Dictionary of Alternative-Medicine Methods, by Priorities for Health editor Jack Raso, M.S., R.D.
Hyperlink: http://www.canoe.ca/AltmedDictionary/a.html

Aromics
Alternative names: aromics program
Source: The Canoe version of A Dictionary of Alternative-Medicine Methods, by Priorities for Health editor Jack Raso, M.S., R.D.
Hyperlink: http://www.canoe.ca/AltmedDictionary/a.html

Cosmetic aromatherapy
Source: The Canoe version of A Dictionary of Alternative-Medicine Methods, by Priorities for Health editor Jack Raso, M.S., R.D.
Hyperlink: http://www.canoe.ca/AltmedDictionary/c.html

DreamLearning
Source: The Canoe version of A Dictionary of Alternative-Medicine Methods, by Priorities for Health editor Jack Raso, M.S., R.D.
Hyperlink: http://www.canoe.ca/AltmedDictionary/d.html

Facial Rejuvenation
Source: The Canoe version of A Dictionary of Alternative-Medicine Methods, by Priorities for Health editor Jack Raso, M.S., R.D.
Hyperlink: http://www.canoe.ca/AltmedDictionary/f.html

Healtheology
Source: The Canoe version of A Dictionary of Alternative-Medicine Methods, by Priorities for Health editor Jack Raso, M.S., R.D.
Hyperlink: http://www.canoe.ca/AltmedDictionary/h.html

Holiday aromatherapy
Source: The Canoe version of A Dictionary of Alternative-Medicine Methods, by Priorities for Health editor Jack Raso, M.S., R.D.
Hyperlink: http://www.canoe.ca/AltmedDictionary/h.html

Magical aromatherapy
Source: The Canoe version of A Dictionary of Alternative-Medicine Methods, by Priorities for Health editor Jack Raso, M.S., R.D.
Hyperlink: http://www.canoe.ca/AltmedDictionary/m.html

Massage aromatherapy
Source: The Canoe version of A Dictionary of Alternative-Medicine Methods, by
Priorities for Health editor Jack Raso, M.S., R.D.
Hyperlink: http://www.canoe.ca/AltmedDictionary/m.html

Odyssey Massage
Source: The Canoe version of A Dictionary of Alternative-Medicine Methods, by
Priorities for Health editor Jack Raso, M.S., R.D.
Hyperlink: http://www.canoe.ca/AltmedDictionary/o.html

Olfactory aromatherapy
Source: The Canoe version of A Dictionary of Alternative-Medicine Methods, by
Priorities for Health editor Jack Raso, M.S., R.D.
Hyperlink: http://www.canoe.ca/AltmedDictionary/o.html

Paraherbalism
Source: The Canoe version of A Dictionary of Alternative-Medicine Methods, by
Priorities for Health editor Jack Raso, M.S., R.D.
Hyperlink: http://www.canoe.ca/AltmedDictionary/p.html

Phytoaromatherapy
Source: The Canoe version of A Dictionary of Alternative-Medicine Methods, by
Priorities for Health editor Jack Raso, M.S., R.D.
Hyperlink: http://www.canoe.ca/AltmedDictionary/p.html

Raindrop Therapy
Source: The Canoe version of A Dictionary of Alternative-Medicine Methods, by
Priorities for Health editor Jack Raso, M.S., R.D.
Hyperlink: http://www.canoe.ca/AltmedDictionary/r.html

Subtle Aromatherapy
Source: The Canoe version of A Dictionary of Alternative-Medicine Methods, by
Priorities for Health editor Jack Raso, M.S., R.D.
Hyperlink: http://www.canoe.ca/AltmedDictionary/s.html

Swedish Massage Therapy
Source: The Canoe version of A Dictionary of Alternative-Medicine Methods, by
Priorities for Health editor Jack Raso, M.S., R.D.
Hyperlink: http://www.canoe.ca/AltmedDictionary/s.html

Tai Chi
Source: Integrative Medicine Communications; www.drkoop.com

Vibrational medicine
Alternative names: energetic medicine energetics medicine energy medicine subtle-
energy medicine vibrational healing vibrational therapies
Source: The Canoe version of A Dictionary of Alternative-Medicine Methods, by
Priorities for Health editor Jack Raso, M.S., R.D.
Hyperlink: http://www.canoe.ca/AltmedDictionary/v.html

- **Herbs and Supplements**

    English Lavendar
    Source: Integrative Medicine Communications; www.drkoop.com

    French Lavendar
    Source: Integrative Medicine Communications; www.drkoop.com

    Lavandula
    Alternative names: Lavender; Lavandula sp.
    Source: Alternative Medicine Foundation, Inc. www.amfoundation.org

    Lavandula angustifolia
    Source: Integrative Medicine Communications; www.drkoop.com

    Lavender
    Alternative names: Lavandula officinalis
    Source: Healthnotes, Inc. www.healthnotes.com

    Lavender
    Alternative names: Lavandula angustifolia, English Lavendar, French Lavendar
    Source: Integrative Medicine Communications; www.drkoop.com

    Lavender
    Source: WholeHealthMD.com, LLC. www.wholehealthmd.com
    Hyperlink:
    http://www.wholehealthmd.com/refshelf/substances_view/0,1525,799,00.html

    Rosmarinus
    Alternative names: Rosemary; Rosmarinus officinalis L.
    Source: Alternative Medicine Foundation, Inc. www.amfoundation.org

    Valeriana
    Alternative names: Valerian; Valeriana officinalis
    Source: Alternative Medicine Foundation, Inc. www.amfoundation.org

General References

A good place to find general background information on CAM is the National Library of Medicine. It has prepared within the MEDLINEplus system an information topic page dedicated to complementary and alternative medicine. To access this page, go to the MEDLINEplus site at **http://www.nlm.nih.gov/medlineplus/alternativemedicine.html**. This Web site provides a general overview of various topics and can lead to a number of general sources.

CHAPTER 4. PATENTS ON AROMATHERAPY

Overview

Patents can be physical innovations (e.g. chemicals, pharmaceuticals, medical equipment) or processes (e.g. treatments or diagnostic procedures). The United States Patent and Trademark Office defines a patent as a grant of a property right to the inventor, issued by the Patent and Trademark Office.[5] Patents, therefore, are intellectual property. For the United States, the term of a new patent is 20 years from the date when the patent application was filed. If the inventor wishes to receive economic benefits, it is likely that the invention will become commercially available within 20 years of the initial filing. It is important to understand, therefore, that an inventor's patent does not indicate that a product or service is or will be commercially available. The patent implies only that the inventor has "the right to exclude others from making, using, offering for sale, or selling" the invention in the United States. While this relates to U.S. patents, similar rules govern foreign patents.

In this chapter, we show you how to locate information on patents and their inventors. If you find a patent that is particularly interesting to you, contact the inventor or the assignee for further information. **IMPORTANT NOTE:** When following the search strategy described below, you may discover non-medical patents that use the generic term "aromatherapy" (or a synonym) in their titles. To accurately reflect the results that you might find while conducting research on aromatherapy, we have not necessarily excluded non-medical patents in this bibliography.

Patents on Aromatherapy

By performing a patent search focusing on aromatherapy, you can obtain information such as the title of the invention, the names of the inventor(s), the assignee(s) or the company that owns or controls the patent, a short abstract that summarizes the patent, and a few excerpts from the description of the patent. The abstract of a patent tends to be more technical in nature, while the description is often written for the public. Full patent descriptions contain much more information than is presented here (e.g. claims, references, figures, diagrams, etc.). We will tell you how to obtain this information later in the chapter. The following is an

---

[5] Adapted from the United States Patent and Trademark Office:
http://www.uspto.gov/web/offices/pac/doc/general/whatis.htm.

example of the type of information that you can expect to obtain from a patent search on aromatherapy:

- **Aromatherapy mats for pets**

  Inventor(s): Licciardo; Rochine (Buchannon, WV)

  Assignee(s): International Marketing Corp. (Westville, NJ)

  Patent Number: 6,173,675

  Date filed: November 12, 1998

  Abstract: The invention is a mattress, mat or bed for animals comprising a soft and comfortable mat which-contains aromatherapy herbs having volatile components which aid and enhance certain behaviors in cats and dogs when laid upon. The mat is constructed with layers of soft fiber filling material and herbs are arranged between the layers and an outer cover of the mat. Preferably the filling material are of such a nature as to aid in the confinement and control of the herb material, while allowing for the full effect of the mixture of the herbs to be obtained. The scent and volatile effects of the herbs are able to emerge through the layers of the filling material and be inhaled by the pet to render the desired behavior.

  Excerpt(s): The invention is related to aromatherapy for animals and more particularly to pet mats filled with aromatic herbs. In the pet accessory industry several types of pet beds are available. Most commonly pet beds are designed simply for the comfort of a cat or a dog, although other beds or mats have deodorizing effects or insect repelling effects. These beds are stuffed with a variety of materials such as wood shavings, powdered insecticides, or other materials suitable to achieve the effects of deodorizing the pet bed or repelling fleas or ticks therefrom. Unknown to pet beds are those which provide the benefits of aromatherapy which humans have come to enjoy and to use therapeutically. Catnip toys have been used to provide a cat with a naturally scented toy which has a appealing odor to a cat and promotes feline activity with the toy. However, until now, there has not been known any toy or pet bed which will calm a cat or a dog or alter specific behavior patterns.

  Web site: http://www.delphion.com/details?pn=US06173675__

- **Aromatherapy scent dispenser having casing with living hinge attached snap fit lid**

  Inventor(s): Bruckner; Tony A. (P.O. Box 297, Clinton, AR 72031), Bruckner; James V. (P.O. Box 297, Clinton, AR 72031), Gurnsey; Robert F. (P.O. Box 297, Clinton, AR 72031)

  Assignee(s): none reported

  Patent Number: 6,102,300

  Date filed: May 3, 1999

  Abstract: A pocket size aromatherapy scent dispenser includes a flat casing defining a narrow cavity, a lid formed by an upper portion of the casing and a living hinge extending across the casing below the upper portion and pivotally connecting the lid to a remainder portion of the casing such that the lid can pivot about the living hinge between opened and closed positions relative to the remainder portion of the casing. The lid in the opened position is pivoted away from the remainder portion of the casing and opens an upper portion of the narrow cavity above the living hinge to an external environment. The lid in the closed position is disposed adjacent to the remainder portion of the casing and closes the upper portion of the cavity to the external environment. A piece of absorbent material carrying an aroma-producing substance is contained within the narrow cavity and has an upper portion partially exposed to the external environment when the lid is in the opened position such that a scent is produced that escapes to the external environment. A flat insert plate is disposed within narrow the cavity of the casing and contacts the upper portion of the piece of material. The insert plate partially exposes the upper portion of the piece of material to the external environment when the lid is in the opened position.

Excerpt(s): The present invention generally relates to devices carrying odoriferous material for dispensing scents and, more particularly, is concerned with a pocket size aromatherapy scent dispenser having a casing with an upper portion forming a living hinge attached snap fit lid. Aromatherapy is a natural, drug-free treatment for the human body which has been found to be significantly effective in relieving the discomforts of many health-related complaints. Aromatherapy is derived from an ancient practice of using natural plant essences to treat illness and enhance health. This ancient practice uses pure essential oils extracted from a wide assortment of natural botanicals. It is believed that these oils found in plants, flowers, fruit, bark and roots provide scents that can restore a healthy balance of the body, mind and spirit. When aromatic molecules are inhaled, they are believed to make contact with nerve-receptacle bundles found at the top of the nasal cavity. When the aromatic essence contacts these nerves, they send signals that result in brain activity. These responses have been observed through brain scans and other diagnostic technologies. Aromatherapy applies to the delicate blending of these oils to treat specific symptoms. Each individual essence has distinct therapeutic qualities.

Web site: http://www.delphion.com/details?pn=US06102300__

- **Floral preservative and aromatherapy apparatus and method**

Inventor(s): Hamley; Robert J. (663 Main St., Hunter, NY 12442)

Assignee(s): none reported

Patent Number: 6,258,748

Date filed: October 27, 1999

Abstract: To preserve flowers and provide aromatherapy, low temperature paraffin is heated to a liquid state of approximately 130 degrees Fahrenheit. A floral nutrient and preservative such as sugar is then added to the low temperature paraffin. Optionally, scents and/or color dyes are also added. The heads of flowers to be preserved are then dipped in this paraffin mixture for one to three seconds and thereafter allowed to dry. The flower can then be used immediately, or optionally hung upside down for one to three weeks prior to use to further improve shelf life.

Excerpt(s): This invention relates to the field of floral preservatives, and specifically, to a device and method used to preserve cut flowers well beyond their ordinary shelf life. Flowers have long been a special gift for birthdays, anniversaries, weddings, and many other special occasions. However, the gift of flowers only lasts for a short time. Within a few short days or weeks, cut flowers wilt and die unless they have been properly preserved. Over time, various approaches to preserving flowers have been developed. These include freeze drying, hang drying, use of silica gels and sand mixtures, and spraying with the various compounds such as polyurethane, hairspray, and shellac. However, none of these approaches is fully satisfactory in terms of the shelf life achieved, the ability to achieve a lasting, pleasant aroma, and/or providing suitable coloration.

Web site: http://www.delphion.com/details?pn=US06258748___

- **Method and appratus for aromatherapy shower**

Inventor(s): Yekutiely; Barak (1278 Wellington Ave., Teaneck, NJ 07666), Yekutiely; David (24 Sheshet Hayamim St., Ramat Hasharon 47247, IL)

Assignee(s): none reported

Patent Number: 6,581,220

Date filed: April 30, 2001

Abstract: A method for aromatherapy including recirculating shower water on a body of a bather, the shower water including at least one aromatherapy substance.

Excerpt(s): The present invention relates generally to aromatherapy and particularly to shower apparatus and methods for aromatherapy. Aromatherapy encompasses a variety of methods for delivering therapeutic benefits of essential oils or base oils of aromatic botanical extracts to the body. One type of aromatherapy involves mixing the aromatic extracts with water for bathing. Bathing with aromatic extracts is well known to provide many types of medicinal benefits. For example, therapeutic bath salts are well known for the relaxation of muscles, elimination or reduction of muscle spasms, and for the overall enhancement of a person's skin and mood. Examples of aromatic botanical extracts used in aromatherapy include, but are not limited to, jojoba oil (a base oil that has a chemical makeup very similar to the naturally occurring sebum in skin), rosewood oil, ylang-ylang oil, lavender oil, patchouli oil and grape seed extract. A bather generally mixes the aromatic extracts with water in a bathtub, and soaks in the tub for a period of time. By resting in the tub, the user accrues the combined benefits of external therapy and internal therapy, such as soothing or relaxing the body, or conditioning or otherwise improving the health of skin, to name a few. Aromatherapy showers are also known. For example, U.S. Pat. Nos. 5,915,622 to Foote and 5,957,379 to McMorrow, et al. both describe shower apparatus for delivering aromatic extracts in a water stream to a person taking a shower. These patents deal with the problem of mixing aromatic botanical extracts with mineral salts in a water stream. The problem is that if botanical extracts are exposed to mineral salts for a prolonged period of time, the mineral salts may cause oxidation of the extracts. This oxidation of the extracts eliminates a majority of the value and benefit of the aromatic character of the extracts.

Web site: http://www.delphion.com/details?pn=US06581220___

- **PMS defense: an aromatherapy compound for the relief of symptoms of premenstrual syndrome**

Inventor(s): Mannella; Lenore C. (177 Riverside Ave., STE F, Newport Beach, CA 92663)

Assignee(s): none reported

Patent Number: 6,322,823

Date filed: May 27, 1999

Abstract: This invention is directed to an Aromatherapy compound to combat symptoms of Premenstrual Syndrome. It uniquely comprises an externally applied compound consisting of "essential oils" (highly concentrated oils extracted from plant cells for use in natural, therapeutic applications) that aid in the relief or reduction of symptoms of PMS. The compound preferably comprises equal proportions of essential oil of geranium, essential oil of clary sage, and essential oil of orange. The compound can be used "neat" (directly on the skin), however, the preferred embodiment is to add the compound to a "carrier" (a base for diluting the Aromatherapy compound) such as lotion or vegetable oil. The preferred formula is approximately 3 milliliters essential oil (1milliliter of geranium, 1 milliliter of clary sage, and 1 milliliter of orange) blended in 120 milliliters of carrier.

Excerpt(s): This invention is directed to an Aromatherapy compound using a unique combination of natural oils extracted from plant cells to combat symptoms of Premenstrual Syndrome. Natural health care companies supply female consumers with a variety of products that purportedly reduce symptoms of PMS. These products may be in the form of vitamin supplementation or herbal compounds, as in U.S. Pat. No. 5,707,630 to Morrow (1998), and more broadly cite relief of ". PMS through menopausal symptoms.". U.S. Pat. No. 5,565,199 to Page & Rector-Page (1996), provides a method of synthesizing natural substitutes for progesterone and estrogen from herbaceous plants, and is taken in capsule form or applied topically. This product targets hormonal replacement associated with menopausal symptoms.

Web site: http://www.delphion.com/details?pn=US06322823__

Patent Applications on Aromatherapy

As of December 2000, U.S. patent applications are open to public viewing.[6] Applications are patent requests which have yet to be granted. (The process to achieve a patent can take several years.) The following patent applications have been filed since December 2000 relating to aromatherapy:

- **Aromatherapy footwear**

  Inventor(s): Freeman, Cindy N. (Calabasas, CA), Nunes, Catherine L. (Los Altos, CA)

  Correspondence: Mandel & Adriano; Suite 710; 55 S. Lake Avenue; Pasadena; CA; 91101; US

  Patent Application Number: 20030009138

  Date filed: June 4, 2002

  Abstract: The present invention is footwear and footwear components including insole pads, inserts and liners containing plant-derived essential oils and/or dried plant products applied to or constructed within the footwear and footwear components to deliver the comfort, disinfectant and/or therapeutic benefits of aromatherapy through direct contact with the wearer's feet with the volatile components of the plant derived oils and/or plant products.

  Excerpt(s): This application claims priority to provisional application, U.S. Serial No. 60/295,730, filed Jun. 4, 2001, the contents of which are hereby incorporated by reference in their entirety into this application. This invention relates to aromatherapy, and in particular to the application of essential oils or volatile plant material to human feet through footwear and/or footwear components, to increase comfort and provide

---

6 This has been a common practice outside the United States prior to December 2000.

therapeutic benefits. In the footwear business, the focus has been on improving comfort and performance by changing the shape, fabric and design, including varying the materials and technology that provide padding and cushioning of the feet of the wearer. Most inventions have heretofore concerned developing processes of molding and contouring the innersoles and arch position of the footwear, evolving padding elements (such as air or gel), or increasing the air circulation within the shoe or footpad.

Web site: http://appft1.uspto.gov/netahtml/PTO/search-bool.html

- **Cleansing compositions with milk protein and aromatherapy**

Inventor(s): Piterski, Catherine A. (River Vale, NJ), Riccardi, Grace; (Hoboken, NJ)

Correspondence: CHARLES N.J. RUGGIERO, ESQ. OHLANDT, GREELEY, RUGGIERO & PERLE, L.L.P. ONE LANDMARK SQUARE; 10th FLOOR; STAMFORD; CT; 06901-2682; US

Patent Application Number: 20020177535

Date filed: March 13, 2002

Abstract: A mild foaming cleanser composition is provided. The cleanser composition has a surfactant system, a moisturizer system, an aromatherapy system and a solvent system. The moisturizer system further includes a milk protein. In addition, the cleanser composition may also include an emulsifier, preservative, pH adjusting agent, thickening agent, emollient, opacifying agent, fragrance, or any combinations thereof.

Excerpt(s): This application is a Continuation-In-Part of U.S. application Ser. No. 10/067,187, filed on Feb. 2, 2002, which claims priority from U.S. Provisional Patent Application Serial No. 60/266,828, filed on Feb. 6, 2001. The present invention relates to cleansing compositions. More particularly, the present invention relates to cleansing compositions for infant and toddler use that have a moisturizer system containing a milk protein for nourishing the skin and an aromatherapy system for promoting calming effect to the user. Typically, baby cleansers have a fairly high level of one or more mild cleansing agents. However, many cleansers clean skin and hair at the expense of drying out or stripping moisture from the skin and/or hair. A conditioner may be included in the cleanser composition for conditioning the skin and/or hair. Most conditioning agents are substantive. Substantive agents adhere to the skin to provide a conditioning effect, thereby causing irritation to sensitive membranes, such as those found in the eye. Thus, substantive compositions are not desirable for use in compositions used for bathing infants or toddlers.

Web site: http://appft1.uspto.gov/netahtml/PTO/search-bool.html

- **Combined aromatherapy air diffuser with Ionizer**

Inventor(s): Dotan, Simon; (Netanya, IL)

Correspondence: Home Care Technologies Ltd; Att: SIMON DOTAN; 45 Pinchas Rossen St. TEL-AVIV; 69512; IL

Patent Application Number: 20010032000

Date filed: December 5, 2000

Abstract: A device, combining the prominent Aromatherapy treatment, together with ionizing.The system creates combined molecules of etheric oil and O.sub.3, loaded with static electrical charge.The procedure is done by airflow, carrying molecules of various kinds of etheric oils.The loaded airflow, with etheric oil molecules, passes by a metal grid, which creates O.sub.3 molecules at its edges. The O.sub.3 molecules are gravitated to the etheric oil molecules that flow nearby, and creating a new molecule. These new molecules are loaded with a static electrical charge, being formed from the connection with the O.sub.3 molecule.LED system, having the homogenous wavelength, is installed in the front side of the device, having a focus at 50-mm. approx. in order to heat up the treated area, and by this to allow a better penetration of the etheric oil.

Excerpt(s): This invention relates to a device that actually operates in three different modes, usually done by a separate device for each mode of action. Said proposed device not only that it does these three separate modes of action, but also, due to the fact that it does the air diffusing prior to the ionization, it causes the air stream that contains inside it the free etheric oil molecules, to gather with the free O.sub.3 molecules that are created throughout the way, by the ionization system. Transferring the static charge to the etheric oil molecules intensifies their chemical reaction, while being in contact with any living tissue whatsoever. The device additional uniqueness is that later on, once it is in contact with the living tissue, this tissue has already been pre-heated by the focused lamps system, which is located in the front side of the device. This system stimulates the blood circulation in the tissue, so by the time the loaded air stream arrives; its absorption in the tissue is much more effectively. LED light system, having a coherent wavelength, such as LED 1, is pointed towards a focusing point located in the front side of said device, around 50 mm. at point 9. Each lamp has an optic lens, lens 16, for concentrating the light beam.

Web site: http://appft1.uspto.gov/netahtml/PTO/search-bool.html

- **Disposable personal aromatherapy mask kit**

  Inventor(s): Dyer, Sally E. (Hilton Head Island, SC)

  Correspondence: ROGER M. RATHBUN; 13 MARGARITA COURT; HILTON HEAD ISLAND; SC; 29926; US

  Patent Application Number: 20030047186

  Date filed: August 8, 2002

  Abstract: An aromatherapy inhalation kit providing portable, disposable and immediate therapy. The kit comprises a vial having a capacity of about 2 ml. pre-filled with one application of pre-blended, predetermined quantity and diluted essential oil, a cone-type mask of paper fiber to which the oil blend is applied; and a heavy weight paper folder to hold the mask and vial in the protective folder. At use, the contents of the vial are dispersed onto the outside surface of the mask. The mask is then worn over the user's nose and mouth and the user inhales the vapors for twenty to thirty minutes to enhance the user's mood and/or condition. The kit is small enough to carry in an automobile glove compartment, a backpack, a purse or a pocket. Since its administration does not rely upon electrical power, it is convenient to use at any time or in any location.

  Excerpt(s): The present patent application is based upon Provisional Patent Application Serial No. 60/318,587, filed Sep. 8, 2001 and entitled "Disposable Personal Aromatherapy Mask Kit". The present invention relates to aromatherapy, and, more particularly, to an improved method of the administration of diluted essential oils to a person through the process of inhalation, and to a kit that can be used to carry out the administration of aromatherapy. Aromatherapy is therapy using essential oils in a variety of ways and for a number of purposes. Essential oils are the volatile, organic constituents of fragrant plant matter, and they contribute to both flavor and fragrance. When distilled for plants, the essential oils become concentrated 100 fold or more, so certain properties become very pronounced in the oils.

Web site: http://appft1.uspto.gov/netahtml/PTO/search-bool.html

- **Method and appratus for aromatherapy shower**

  Inventor(s): Yekutiely, David; (Ramat Hasharon, IL), Yekutiely, Barak; (Teaneck, NJ)

  Correspondence: Dekel Patent Ltd. Apt.4; 12 HaEgoz Street; Rehovot; IL

  Patent Application Number: 20020158138

  Date filed: April 30, 2001

  Abstract: A method for aromatherapy including recirculating shower water on a body of a bather, the shower water including at least one aromatherapy substance.

  Excerpt(s): The present invention relates generally to aromatherapy and particularly to shower apparatus and methods for aromatherapy. Aromatherapy encompasses a variety of methods for delivering therapeutic benefits of essential oils or base oils of aromatic botanical extracts to the body. One type of aromatherapy involves mixing the aromatic extracts with water for bathing. Bathing with aromatic extracts is well known to provide many types of medicinal benefits. For example, therapeutic bath salts are well known for the relaxation of muscles, elimination or reduction of muscle spasms, and for the overall enhancement of a person's skin and mood. Examples of aromatic botanical extracts used in aromatherapy include, but are not limited to, jojoba oil (a base oil that has a chemical makeup very similar to the naturally occurring sebum in skin), rosewood oil, ylang-ylang oil, lavender oil, patchouli oil and grape seed extract. A bather generally mixes the aromatic extracts with water in a bathtub, and soaks in the tub for a period of time. By resting in the tub, the user accrues the combined benefits of external therapy and internal therapy, such as soothing or relaxing the body, or conditioning or otherwise improving the health of skin, to name a few. Aromatherapy showers are also known. For example, U.S. Pat. No. 5,915,622 to Foote and U.S. Pat. No. 5,957,379 to McMorrow, et al. both describe shower apparatus for delivering aromatic extracts in a water stream to a person taking a shower. These patents deal with the problem of mixing aromatic botanical extracts with mineral salts in a water stream. The problem is that if botanical extracts are exposed to mineral salts for a prolonged period of time, the mineral salts may cause oxidation of the extracts. This oxidation of the extracts eliminates a majority of the value and benefit of the aromatic character of the extracts.

  Web site: http://appft1.uspto.gov/netahtml/PTO/search-bool.html

Keeping Current

In order to stay informed about patents and patent applications dealing with aromatherapy, you can access the U.S. Patent Office archive via the Internet at the following Web address: **http://www.uspto.gov/patft/index.html**. You will see two broad options: (1) Issued Patent, and (2) Published Applications. To see a list of issued patents, perform the following steps: Under "Issued Patents," click "Quick Search." Then, type "aromatherapy" (or synonyms) into the "Term 1" box. After clicking on the search button, scroll down to see the various patents which have been granted to date on aromatherapy.

You can also use this procedure to view pending patent applications concerning aromatherapy. Simply go back to the following Web address: **http://www.uspto.gov/patft/index.html.** Select "Quick Search" under "Published Applications." Then proceed with the steps listed above.

CHAPTER 5. BOOKS ON AROMATHERAPY

Overview

This chapter provides bibliographic book references relating to aromatherapy. In addition to online booksellers such as **www.amazon.com** and **www.bn.com**, excellent sources for book titles on aromatherapy include the Combined Health Information Database and the National Library of Medicine. Your local medical library also may have these titles available for loan.

Book Summaries: Federal Agencies

The Combined Health Information Database collects various book abstracts from a variety of healthcare institutions and federal agencies. To access these summaries, go directly to the following hyperlink: **http://chid.nih.gov/detail/detail.html**. You will need to use the "Detailed Search" option. To find book summaries, use the drop boxes at the bottom of the search page where "You may refine your search by." Select the dates and language you prefer. For the format option, select "Monograph/Book." Now type "aromatherapy" (or synonyms) into the "For these words:" box. You should check back periodically with this database which is updated every three months. The following is a typical result when searching for books on aromatherapy:

- **Irritable Bowel Syndrome (IBS) and Gastrointestinal Solutions Handbook**

  Source: Encinitas, CA: United Research Publishers. 1997. 232 p.

  Contact: Available from United Research Publishers. Department RB-91, 103 North Coast Highway 101, Encinitas, CA 92024. PRICE: $14.95. ISBN: 096149249X.

  Summary: This book discusses irritable bowel syndrome (IBS) and other gastrointestinal problems and explains how readers can educate themselves, treat problems, and prevent recurrences of these conditions. The author discusses natural, alternative, and medical remedies that can bring relief without the use of drugs. The author also explains how the gastrointestinal system works, why certain foods, activities, and stress cause problems, and why over 20 million Americans deal with IBS and gastrointestinal distress. One chapter in the book discusses other diseases of the digestive tract and notes that they require a doctor's attention but are often easier to treat than IBS. IBS, however, can be individualistic, intermittent, and difficult to treat. The last section reviews some nontraditional helps and ideas that might be of use, including homeopathy, relaxation, hypnotherapy, **aromatherapy,** herbal remedies, and acupuncture. A final chapter lists fat grams and calories for many common foods.

- **Nutrition Almanac. 4th ed**

    Source: New York, NY: McGraw-Hill, 494p., paperback, 1996.

    Summary: This book discusses several aspects of nutrition: nutrition and health, exercise, sources of calories, nutrients, and the role of nutrition in the life cycle. Also included are chapters on alternative therapies such as herbology, **aromatherapy,** and homeopathy.

- **Help, Comfort and Hope After Losing Your Baby in Pregnancy or the First Year**

    Source: Cambridge, MA: Fisher Books/Perseus Books Group. 1997. 294 p.

    Contact: Available from Fisher Books/Perseus Books Group, 11 Cambridge Center, Cambridge, MA 02142. (617) 252-5200 (marketing and editorial), (800) 386-5656 (orders), (303) 449-3356 (Fax), info@perseuspublishing.com (E-mail), http://www.perseuspublishing.com (Web Site). $12.95. ISBN 1-55561-120-6.

    Summary: This book is written for parents who have experienced pregnancy loss or infant death and for the caregivers who are there to support them. The author lost a baby during pregnancy in 1984 and now leads workshops in perinatal bereavement counseling for physicians, nurses, midwives, clergy and other professionals who come in contact with families who have suffered a pregnancy or infant loss. Chapter 1 looks at the legal definition and medical aspects of miscarriage, stillbirth, neonatal death, sudden infant death syndrome (SIDS), and termination of pregnancy. This chapter also discusses the grief and loss associated with adoption and the special grief of single bereaved mothers. Chapter 2 examines the nature of grieving, which usually begins with shock and emotional numbness. In situations in which a miscarriage has occurred and curettage is to be performed to remove the dead embryo or fetus, or if the mother is to undergo vaginal birth, with contractions, of a fully developed baby, she is encouraged to find out what her options are and to make as many decisions as she can on her own. If she is not getting the support and answers she needs from the hospital staff, she should seek out her own support. This chapter also discusses the process of letting go of the fetus or baby; taking one's time to make that decision; ways to facilitate the grief process; and the various scenarios that can occur (e.g., miscarriage in the first 3 months, induced birth of a developed baby who has died, death during or shortly after cesarean birth, and the birth of a seriously ill infant); bonding with the baby; family-centered stillbirth; naming and baptizing the baby; collecting mementos; autopsy and burial decisions; and the need for rituals. Chapter 3 describes the second phase of grief, searching and yearning, which is full of powerful emotions like pain, anger, guilt, fear, despair, and jealousy. This phase usually lasts 4 to 6 months. In this chapter, the author encourages bereaved mothers to acknowledge and express their feelings and provides specific actions and exercises to help them find comfort and relief. This chapter also discusses taking a break from grief, finding consolation, attending a support group, a father's grief, grief and the marital relationship, siblings' grief, and a grandparent's grief. In chapter 4, the author gives bereaved parents suggestions for coping with grief 6 months after the death and beyond. This is when parents have grasped the reality of the death and are slowly adapting to life without their baby. The length of this phase differs from individual to individual. This chapter contains suggestions for nurturing the physical self with proper nutrition, exercise, sleep, and holistic treatments. The author describes the power of visualization, creativity, spirituality, **aromatherapy,** and flower essences in healing from grief; what to do when the grief process stagnates; and when professional help is needed. Chapter 5 looks at the period following the anniversary of the death, a period of closure and new beginnings, including the possibility of having another child. The remaining chapters are intended for those who care for the bereaved. Chapter 6 reviews what the bereaved need and don't need from others during mourning. Chapter 7 is a primer on what health care professionals can do to support and comfort the parents who have miscarried or whose infant has died in the hospital setting. The author describes specific things caretakers can do (i.e., take a photo) and how they can set up a perinatal bereavement team. The chapter also contains 12 pages of guidelines for parents' care after stillbirth, miscarriage, and newborn death. The guidelines address what to do when the mother is admitted to the hospital, during labor and delivery, during postpartum care, and upon discharge. Chapter 8 focuses on what the hospital staff and others can do for the bereaved parents after they leave the hospital. Ideally, followup care should be given by all of the following: the mother's gynecologist or family physician; a visiting nurse, midwife, or doula; a pastor, priest, or rabbi; and a counselor or therapist. This chapter discusses how caregivers can support parents through the four phases of grief and the five tasks of mourners; monitor the health of the bereaved; recognize signs of complicated mourning; and provide care during subsequent pregnancies. Chapter 9 discusses the spiritual care of the bereaved; including the parents' right to have their child baptized, the power of rituals in healing grief, and how clergy can help bereaved parents. Chapter 10 discusses the value of support groups for bereaved parents, how parents can form their own group, the SHARE support group model, and topics for group meetings. Chapter 11 examines dealing with death in childbirth education classes, including how childbirth educators can bring up the topic, how to handle couples who have had a previous loss, what to do when a couple in the class suffers a loss, and how the group and educator can be supportive if that happens. Chapter 12 looks at what funeral directors can do to facilitate the grief process. Appendix 1 presents the rights of parents when a baby dies. Appendix 2 provides questionnaires for assessing the grief of parents and for assessing caregivers' personal experiences with and attitudes toward death and dying. Appendix 3 presents suggestions for meditation; memorial rituals; and readings, prayers, and songs. Appendix 4 is a directory of support organizations, bereavement web sites, publishers of bereavement materials, audiovisual materials, sources of information on therapy, and sources of natural remedies. An extensive bibliography and a list of journals and newsletters complete the book.

Book Summaries: Online Booksellers

Commercial Internet-based booksellers, such as Amazon.com and Barnes&Noble.com, offer summaries which have been supplied by each title's publisher. Some summaries also include customer reviews. Your local bookseller may have access to in-house and commercial databases that index all published books (e.g. Books in Print®). **IMPORTANT NOTE:** Online booksellers typically produce search results for medical and non-medical books. When searching for "aromatherapy" at online booksellers' Web sites, you may discover non-medical books that use the generic term "aromatherapy" (or a synonym) in their titles. The following is indicative of the results you might find when searching for "aromatherapy" (sorted alphabetically by title; follow the hyperlink to view more details at Amazon.com):

- **"Nature's Way" Guide to Aromatherapy** by John Woodruff; ISBN: 1870228154; http://www.amazon.com/exec/obidos/ASIN/1870228154/icongroupinterna

- **"Reader's Digest" Bathing for Health, Beauty and Relaxation: Treatments, Aromatherapy, Ingredients** by Eva Gizowska; ISBN: 0276423968; http://www.amazon.com/exec/obidos/ASIN/0276423968/icongroupinterna

- **25 Aromatherapy Blends for De-Stressing (Storey Country Wisdom Bulletin, A-244)** by Victoria H. Edwards (2000); ISBN: 1580173055; http://www.amazon.com/exec/obidos/ASIN/1580173055/icongroupinterna

- **500 Formulas For Aromatherapy: Mixing Essential Oils for Every Use** by David Schiller, Carol Schiller (Contributor) (1994); ISBN: 0806905840; http://www.amazon.com/exec/obidos/ASIN/0806905840/icongroupinterna

- **556 Aromatherapy Formulas for Mind & Body** by David Schiller, Carol Schiller (2001); ISBN: 0806976314; http://www.amazon.com/exec/obidos/ASIN/0806976314/icongroupinterna

- **A Z Aromatherapy** by Patricia Davis (Author); ISBN: 1566199735; http://www.amazon.com/exec/obidos/ASIN/1566199735/icongroupinterna

- **Advanced Aromatherapy: The Science of Essential Oil Therapy** by Kurt Schnaubelt (1998); ISBN: 0892817437; http://www.amazon.com/exec/obidos/ASIN/0892817437/icongroupinterna

- **All You Wanted to Know About Aromatherapy** by Lalitha Sharma; ISBN: 8120722728; http://www.amazon.com/exec/obidos/ASIN/8120722728/icongroupinterna

- **Alternative Health Therapies: The Complete Guide to Aromatherapy, Massage, and Reflexology** by Denise Whichello Brown, Sandra White (2002); ISBN: 1577172175; http://www.amazon.com/exec/obidos/ASIN/1577172175/icongroupinterna

- **Alternative Health: Aromatherapy (Alternative Health)** by Vivian Lunny; ISBN: 0861019067; http://www.amazon.com/exec/obidos/ASIN/0861019067/icongroupinterna

- **An Introductory Guide to Aromatherapy** by Louise Tucker; ISBN: 1903348013; http://www.amazon.com/exec/obidos/ASIN/1903348013/icongroupinterna

- **Ancient Aromatherapy**; ISBN: 7215981215; http://www.amazon.com/exec/obidos/ASIN/7215981215/icongroupinterna

- **Aromaterapia Para Amantes/Aromatherapy/Lovers** by Feller Tara (1998); ISBN: 9684039948; http://www.amazon.com/exec/obidos/ASIN/9684039948/icongroupinterna

- **Aromatherapy** by Julia Lawless (2002); ISBN: 0007131089; http://www.amazon.com/exec/obidos/ASIN/0007131089/icongroupinterna

- **Aromatherapy** by Gill Martin; ISBN: 0356171132; http://www.amazon.com/exec/obidos/ASIN/0356171132/icongroupinterna

- **Aromatherapy** by Consumer Guide (Editor), et al; ISBN: 0451199073; http://www.amazon.com/exec/obidos/ASIN/0451199073/icongroupinterna

- **Aromatherapy** by Micheline Arcier, Fiona Pragoff (Photographer); ISBN: 0600575608; http://www.amazon.com/exec/obidos/ASIN/0600575608/icongroupinterna

- **Aromatherapy** by Julie Sadler; ISBN: 0706369599; http://www.amazon.com/exec/obidos/ASIN/0706369599/icongroupinterna

- **Aromatherapy** by Liz Earle; ISBN: 0752205587;
  http://www.amazon.com/exec/obidos/ASIN/0752205587/icongroupinterna

- **Aromatherapy** (2003); ISBN: 0752588796;
  http://www.amazon.com/exec/obidos/ASIN/0752588796/icongroupinterna

- **Aromatherapy** by Victoria Hyun; ISBN: 0762411317;
  http://www.amazon.com/exec/obidos/ASIN/0762411317/icongroupinterna

- **Aromatherapy** by Joanna Drew (Editor); ISBN: 0785804463;
  http://www.amazon.com/exec/obidos/ASIN/0785804463/icongroupinterna

- **Aromatherapy** by Ann Ross Paterson (1996); ISBN: 0863155952;
  http://www.amazon.com/exec/obidos/ASIN/0863155952/icongroupinterna

- **Aromatherapy** by Judith Jackson; ISBN: 0863182216;
  http://www.amazon.com/exec/obidos/ASIN/0863182216/icongroupinterna

- **Aromatherapy** by Jan Balkam; ISBN: 1856052311;
  http://www.amazon.com/exec/obidos/ASIN/1856052311/icongroupinterna

- **Aromatherapy** by Nerys Purchon (1995); ISBN: 1856276848;
  http://www.amazon.com/exec/obidos/ASIN/1856276848/icongroupinterna

- **Aromatherapy** by Marjorie Shakespeare; ISBN: 1858219167;
  http://www.amazon.com/exec/obidos/ASIN/1858219167/icongroupinterna

- **AROMATHERAPY**; ISBN: 3576100806;
  http://www.amazon.com/exec/obidos/ASIN/3576100806/icongroupinterna

- **Aromatherapy - a Nurses Guide** by Ann Percival (1995); ISBN: 1899308040;
  http://www.amazon.com/exec/obidos/ASIN/1899308040/icongroupinterna

- **Aromatherapy - a Nurses Guide for Women** by Ann Percival (1996); ISBN: 1899308121;
  http://www.amazon.com/exec/obidos/ASIN/1899308121/icongroupinterna

- **Aromatherapy - An A to Z** by Patricia Davis (1999); ISBN: 0852072953;
  http://www.amazon.com/exec/obidos/ASIN/0852072953/icongroupinterna

- **Aromatherapy - Beauty Therapy Basics** by Helen McGuinness; ISBN: 034067993X;
  http://www.amazon.com/exec/obidos/ASIN/034067993X/icongroupinterna

- **Aromatherapy - for Healthy Legs and Feet** by Christine Westwood (1995); ISBN: 1899308024;
  http://www.amazon.com/exec/obidos/ASIN/1899308024/icongroupinterna

- **Aromatherapy - Stress Management** by Christine Westwood (1998); ISBN: 0951772368;
  http://www.amazon.com/exec/obidos/ASIN/0951772368/icongroupinterna

- **Aromatherapy & Complementary Therapies**; ISBN: 1842050281;
  http://www.amazon.com/exec/obidos/ASIN/1842050281/icongroupinterna

- **Aromatherapy & Subtle Energy Techniques: Compassionate Healing With Essential Oils** by Joni Loughran, Ruah Bull (2000); ISBN: 1583940154;
  http://www.amazon.com/exec/obidos/ASIN/1583940154/icongroupinterna

- **Aromatherapy (Collins Gems Series)** by Lucinda Deacon-Davis, Harpercollins (2001); ISBN: 0007101465;
  http://www.amazon.com/exec/obidos/ASIN/0007101465/icongroupinterna

- **Aromatherapy (Complementary Health)** by Vivan Lunny, Vivian Lunny; ISBN: 0765199556;
  http://www.amazon.com/exec/obidos/ASIN/0765199556/icongroupinterna

- **Aromatherapy (Headway Lifeguides)** by Denise Brown; ISBN: 0340559500;
  http://www.amazon.com/exec/obidos/ASIN/0340559500/icongroupinterna

- **Aromatherapy (Health)** (1996); ISBN: 075251301X;
  http://www.amazon.com/exec/obidos/ASIN/075251301X/icongroupinterna

- **Aromatherapy (Naturally Better)** by Anna Selby, Peter Albright (Editor); ISBN: 0028608321;
  http://www.amazon.com/exec/obidos/ASIN/0028608321/icongroupinterna

- **Aromatherapy (Penguin Health)** by Robert Tisserand; ISBN: 0140096833;
  http://www.amazon.com/exec/obidos/ASIN/0140096833/icongroupinterna

- **Aromatherapy (Pocket Healing Books, 1)** by Kevin Hudson (2000); ISBN: 965494104X;
  http://www.amazon.com/exec/obidos/ASIN/965494104X/icongroupinterna

- **Aromatherapy (The Practical Health Series)** by Penny Rich; ISBN: 0765198126;
  http://www.amazon.com/exec/obidos/ASIN/0765198126/icongroupinterna

- **AROMATHERAPY (THORSONS)** by Raymond Lautie; ISBN: 0722511450;
  http://www.amazon.com/exec/obidos/ASIN/0722511450/icongroupinterna

- **Aromatherapy (Woodland Health Ser)** by Woodland Publishing Staff, Woodland Publishing (1999); ISBN: 1885670729;
  http://www.amazon.com/exec/obidos/ASIN/1885670729/icongroupinterna

- **Aromatherapy 101** by Karen Downes (2000); ISBN: 1561706922;
  http://www.amazon.com/exec/obidos/ASIN/1561706922/icongroupinterna

- **Aromatherapy 14 Day Beauty** by Tisserand; ISBN: 0091782473;
  http://www.amazon.com/exec/obidos/ASIN/0091782473/icongroupinterna

- **Aromatherapy and Massage** by Allison England (2000); ISBN: 0091822750;
  http://www.amazon.com/exec/obidos/ASIN/0091822750/icongroupinterna

- **Aromatherapy and Massage for Mother and Baby** by Allison England; ISBN: 0892818980;
  http://www.amazon.com/exec/obidos/ASIN/0892818980/icongroupinterna

- **Aromatherapy and Massage for People with Learning Difficulties** by Helen Sanderson, et al (1991); ISBN: 0951817205;
  http://www.amazon.com/exec/obidos/ASIN/0951817205/icongroupinterna

- **Aromatherapy and Massage: Achieving Health and Well-Being the Natural Way with Simple Massage Techniques and Aromatic Treatments** by Sarah Porter, et al; ISBN: 184038204X;
  http://www.amazon.com/exec/obidos/ASIN/184038204X/icongroupinterna

- **Aromatherapy and the Mind** by Julia Lawless; ISBN: 0722529279;
  http://www.amazon.com/exec/obidos/ASIN/0722529279/icongroupinterna

- **Aromatherapy and You Guide to Natural Skin Care** by Alexandra Avery (Author); ISBN: 0963075020;
  http://www.amazon.com/exec/obidos/ASIN/0963075020/icongroupinterna

- **Aromatherapy and Your Emotions** by Shirley Price; ISBN: 0722538626;
  http://www.amazon.com/exec/obidos/ASIN/0722538626/icongroupinterna

- **Aromatherapy Anointing Oils: Spiritual Blessings, Ceremonies, and Affirmations** by Joni Keim Loughran, et al; ISBN: 1583940456; http://www.amazon.com/exec/obidos/ASIN/1583940456/icongroupinterna

- **Aromatherapy A-Z (Hay House Lifestyles)** by Connie Higley, et al; ISBN: 156170489X; http://www.amazon.com/exec/obidos/ASIN/156170489X/icongroupinterna

- **Aromatherapy Baby Book** by Marion Del Gaudio Mak (1998); ISBN: 1899308180; http://www.amazon.com/exec/obidos/ASIN/1899308180/icongroupinterna

- **Aromatherapy Basics** by Carol Schiller, et al; ISBN: 0806997850; http://www.amazon.com/exec/obidos/ASIN/0806997850/icongroupinterna

- **Aromatherapy Blends and Remedies: Over 800 Recipes for Everyday Use** by Franzesca Watson, Christine Lane (Illustrator) (1996); ISBN: 0722532229; http://www.amazon.com/exec/obidos/ASIN/0722532229/icongroupinterna

- **Aromatherapy Box Set (Health)**; ISBN: 0752513117; http://www.amazon.com/exec/obidos/ASIN/0752513117/icongroupinterna

- **Aromatherapy Decoder** by Dynamo House; ISBN: 0949266345; http://www.amazon.com/exec/obidos/ASIN/0949266345/icongroupinterna

- **Aromatherapy During Your Pregnancy** by Frances R. Clifford, Lyn Greenwood (Compiler) (1997); ISBN: 0852073127; http://www.amazon.com/exec/obidos/ASIN/0852073127/icongroupinterna

- **Aromatherapy for All** by Joanna Trevelyan (2001); ISBN: 1902463471; http://www.amazon.com/exec/obidos/ASIN/1902463471/icongroupinterna

- **Aromatherapy for Animals: Healing Animals with Essential Oils and Plant Extracts** by Caroline Ingraham (2002); ISBN: 1903360064; http://www.amazon.com/exec/obidos/ASIN/1903360064/icongroupinterna

- **Aromatherapy for Babies and Children** by Shirley Price, Penny Price Parr; ISBN: 0722531079; http://www.amazon.com/exec/obidos/ASIN/0722531079/icongroupinterna

- **Aromatherapy for Back Pain** by Leon Chaitow; ISBN: 185833957X; http://www.amazon.com/exec/obidos/ASIN/185833957X/icongroupinterna

- **Aromatherapy for Beauty Therapist Worwood A**; ISBN: 0333741633; http://www.amazon.com/exec/obidos/ASIN/0333741633/icongroupinterna

- **Aromatherapy for common ailments** by Shirley Price; ISBN: 1856750051; http://www.amazon.com/exec/obidos/ASIN/1856750051/icongroupinterna

- **Aromatherapy For Dummies®** by Kathi Keville (Author) (1999); ISBN: 076455171X; http://www.amazon.com/exec/obidos/ASIN/076455171X/icongroupinterna

- **Aromatherapy for Healing the Spirit: A Guide to Restoring Emotional and Mental Balance Through Essential Oils** by Gabriel Mojay; ISBN: 0805044965; http://www.amazon.com/exec/obidos/ASIN/0805044965/icongroupinterna

- **Aromatherapy for Healing the Spirit: Restoring Emotional and Mental Balance with Essential Oils** by Gabriel Mojay (2000); ISBN: 0892818875; http://www.amazon.com/exec/obidos/ASIN/0892818875/icongroupinterna

- **Aromatherapy for Health Professionals** by Shirley Price, et al; ISBN: 0443062102; http://www.amazon.com/exec/obidos/ASIN/0443062102/icongroupinterna

- **Aromatherapy for Health, Beauty, and Well-being** by McGilvery, Reed; ISBN: 1840385642;
http://www.amazon.com/exec/obidos/ASIN/1840385642/icongroupinterna

- **Aromatherapy for Holistic Therapists** by Francesca Gould (2003); ISBN: 0748771026;
http://www.amazon.com/exec/obidos/ASIN/0748771026/icongroupinterna

- **Aromatherapy for Horses** by Caroline Ingraham, Carole Vincer (Illustrator) (1997); ISBN: 187208298X;
http://www.amazon.com/exec/obidos/ASIN/187208298X/icongroupinterna

- **Aromatherapy for Lovers and Dreamers** by Judith White (Editor), et al; ISBN: 0517886677;
http://www.amazon.com/exec/obidos/ASIN/0517886677/icongroupinterna

- **Aromatherapy for Lovers: Essential Recipes for Romance** by Tara Fellner, Mary Sundstrom; ISBN: 1582900469;
http://www.amazon.com/exec/obidos/ASIN/1582900469/icongroupinterna

- **Aromatherapy for Midwifery Practice** by Churchill Livingstone, Tiran; ISBN: 070201978X;
http://www.amazon.com/exec/obidos/ASIN/070201978X/icongroupinterna

- **Aromatherapy for Mind & Body** by David Schiller, Carol Schiller (Contributor) (2001); ISBN: 0806942444;
http://www.amazon.com/exec/obidos/ASIN/0806942444/icongroupinterna

- **Aromatherapy for Mother** by England; ISBN: 009177487X;
http://www.amazon.com/exec/obidos/ASIN/009177487X/icongroupinterna

- **Aromatherapy for Mother & Baby** by Allison England, Lola Borg; ISBN: 0892814861;
http://www.amazon.com/exec/obidos/ASIN/0892814861/icongroupinterna

- **Aromatherapy for Pregnancy and Childbirth (Home Library of Alternative Medicine)** by Margaret, Rgn Fawcett; ISBN: 1852303905;
http://www.amazon.com/exec/obidos/ASIN/1852303905/icongroupinterna

- **Aromatherapy for Sensual Awareness: Care for the Body and Mind With Nature's Essential Oils** by Judith White, et al (1996); ISBN: 0517886669;
http://www.amazon.com/exec/obidos/ASIN/0517886669/icongroupinterna

- **Aromatherapy for the Beauty Therapist: Hairdressing And Beauty Industry Authority/Thomson Learning Series** by Valerie Ann Worwood; ISBN: 1861526636;
http://www.amazon.com/exec/obidos/ASIN/1861526636/icongroupinterna

- **Aromatherapy for the Family** by Kusmirek; ISBN: 0946982066;
http://www.amazon.com/exec/obidos/ASIN/0946982066/icongroupinterna

- **Aromatherapy for the Healthy Child: More Than 300 Natural, Non-Toxic, and Fragrant Essential Oil Blends** by Valerie Ann Worwood (2000); ISBN: 1577310950;
http://www.amazon.com/exec/obidos/ASIN/1577310950/icongroupinterna

- **Aromatherapy for the Whole Person** by W.E. Arnould-Taylor; ISBN: 0859503372;
http://www.amazon.com/exec/obidos/ASIN/0859503372/icongroupinterna

- **Aromatherapy for Travellers: How to Use Essential Oils for Health and Well-Being While Travelling** by Jude Brown; ISBN: 0722531206;
http://www.amazon.com/exec/obidos/ASIN/0722531206/icongroupinterna

- **Aromatherapy for Vibrant Health & Beauty/a Practical A to Z Reference of Aromatherapy Treatments for Health, Skin, and Hair Problems Using Essential** by

Roberta Wilson (1995); ISBN: 0895296276;
http://www.amazon.com/exec/obidos/ASIN/0895296276/icongroupinterna

- **Aromatherapy for Women** by Shirley Price (2004); ISBN: 184215916X;
http://www.amazon.com/exec/obidos/ASIN/184215916X/icongroupinterna

- **Aromatherapy for Women and Children: Pregnancy and Childbirth** by Jane Dye
(1993); ISBN: 0852072260;
http://www.amazon.com/exec/obidos/ASIN/0852072260/icongroupinterna

- **Aromatherapy for Women How to Use Essent** by Maggie Tisserand (Author); ISBN:
0722522606;
http://www.amazon.com/exec/obidos/ASIN/0722522606/icongroupinterna

- **Aromatherapy for Women: A Practical Guide to Essential Oils for Health and Beauty**
by Maggie Tisserand (1996); ISBN: 0892816287;
http://www.amazon.com/exec/obidos/ASIN/0892816287/icongroupinterna

- **Aromatherapy for Women: Aromatic Essential Oils for Natural Healing** by Shirley
Price, Michelle Garrett (Photographer) (2001); ISBN: 0754806707;
http://www.amazon.com/exec/obidos/ASIN/0754806707/icongroupinterna

- **Aromatherapy for You and Your Child: A Personal Guide to Using
Aromatherapy/Aromatherapy Kit Includes 3 Vials of Essences** by Tara Fellner Boles,
Betsy James (Illustrator); ISBN: 0804830436;
http://www.amazon.com/exec/obidos/ASIN/0804830436/icongroupinterna

- **Aromatherapy Fragrance Blending Decoder** by Dynamo House; ISBN: 0949266876;
http://www.amazon.com/exec/obidos/ASIN/0949266876/icongroupinterna

- **Aromatherapy from Provence** by Nelly Grosjean (1994); ISBN: 085207266X;
http://www.amazon.com/exec/obidos/ASIN/085207266X/icongroupinterna

- **Aromatherapy Handbook for Beauty, Hair and Skin Care: A Guide to the Use of
Essential Oils for Beauty and Healing** by Erich Keller; ISBN: 0892814330;
http://www.amazon.com/exec/obidos/ASIN/0892814330/icongroupinterna

- **Aromatherapy Handbook for Beauty, Hair, and Skin Care** by Erich Keller; ISBN:
089281831X;
http://www.amazon.com/exec/obidos/ASIN/089281831X/icongroupinterna

- **Aromatherapy Home Study Mini-Course** by Jonathan Parker; ISBN: 1584000538;
http://www.amazon.com/exec/obidos/ASIN/1584000538/icongroupinterna

- **AROMATHERAPY HOME USE DECODER** by DYNAMO HOUSE; ISBN: 0949266620;
http://www.amazon.com/exec/obidos/ASIN/0949266620/icongroupinterna

- **Aromatherapy in Midwifery** by Burns; ISBN: 0750652918;
http://www.amazon.com/exec/obidos/ASIN/0750652918/icongroupinterna

- **Aromatherapy in Pregnancy and Childbirth** by Jane Dye (1991); ISBN: 0846415364;
http://www.amazon.com/exec/obidos/ASIN/0846415364/icongroupinterna

- **Aromatherapy in the Kitchen: Fragrant Foods for Body, Mind and Spirit** by Melissa
Dale, et al (2002); ISBN: 1580543480;
http://www.amazon.com/exec/obidos/ASIN/1580543480/icongroupinterna

- **Aromatherapy in Your Diet: Discover the Therapeutic Benefits of Everyday Foods** by
Daniele Ryman; ISBN: 074991470X;
http://www.amazon.com/exec/obidos/ASIN/074991470X/icongroupinterna

- **Aromatherapy in Your Diet: How to Enjoy the Health Benefits of Aromatherapy Without Using Essentials Oils** by Daniele Ryman; ISBN: 0425159787; http://www.amazon.com/exec/obidos/ASIN/0425159787/icongroupinterna

- **Aromatherapy Lexicon: The Essential Reference (Lexicon)** by Geoff Lyth, Sue Charles (1997); ISBN: 1899308156; http://www.amazon.com/exec/obidos/ASIN/1899308156/icongroupinterna

- **Aromatherapy Made Easy: Simple Step-By-Step Guide to Using Essential Oils** by Christine Wildwood; ISBN: 0722534523; http://www.amazon.com/exec/obidos/ASIN/0722534523/icongroupinterna

- **Aromatherapy Massage** by Clare Maxwell-Hudson; ISBN: 1564586421; http://www.amazon.com/exec/obidos/ASIN/1564586421/icongroupinterna

- **Aromatherapy Massage Book** by Clare Maxwell-Hudson; ISBN: 067085851X; http://www.amazon.com/exec/obidos/ASIN/067085851X/icongroupinterna

- **Aromatherapy Massage from Head to Toe (Storey Country Wisdom Bulletin, A-254)** by Blair Dils (Editor), et al (2000); ISBN: 1580173012; http://www.amazon.com/exec/obidos/ASIN/1580173012/icongroupinterna

- **Aromatherapy Massage Gift Book**; ISBN: 0751301876; http://www.amazon.com/exec/obidos/ASIN/0751301876/icongroupinterna

- **Aromatherapy Massage: Harnessing the Powers of Essential Oils and Therapeutic Touch Techniques** by Sarah Porter (Editor), et al (2002); ISBN: 1842155571; http://www.amazon.com/exec/obidos/ASIN/1842155571/icongroupinterna

- **Aromatherapy Natural Healing Ess Oil** by COOKSLEY; ISBN: 0130855103; http://www.amazon.com/exec/obidos/ASIN/0130855103/icongroupinterna

- **Aromatherapy Oils: A Complete Guide** by Jeffrey Schiller, et al; ISBN: 0806961120; http://www.amazon.com/exec/obidos/ASIN/0806961120/icongroupinterna

- **Aromatherapy Pack** by Maxwell-Hudson; ISBN: 0751305723; http://www.amazon.com/exec/obidos/ASIN/0751305723/icongroupinterna

- **Aromatherapy Pocketbook** by Kendra Grace; ISBN: 156718183X; http://www.amazon.com/exec/obidos/ASIN/156718183X/icongroupinterna

- **Aromatherapy Scent & Psyche** by Peter Damian, Kate Damian; ISBN: 0892815302; http://www.amazon.com/exec/obidos/ASIN/0892815302/icongroupinterna

- **Aromatherapy Solutions: Essential Oils to Lift the Mind, Body and Spirit** by Veronica Sibley (2003); ISBN: 0600606848; http://www.amazon.com/exec/obidos/ASIN/0600606848/icongroupinterna

- **Aromatherapy Stress Gift Set** by Leon Chaitow, Bramley; ISBN: 185833621X; http://www.amazon.com/exec/obidos/ASIN/185833621X/icongroupinterna

- **Aromatherapy the a Z Guide to Healing With** by Shelagh Rya Masline (Author); ISBN: 1568657846; http://www.amazon.com/exec/obidos/ASIN/1568657846/icongroupinterna

- **Aromatherapy the Essential Beginning** by Gary Young (Author); ISBN: 0964818701; http://www.amazon.com/exec/obidos/ASIN/0964818701/icongroupinterna

- **Aromatherapy Through the Seasons: Restorative Recipes and Sensory Suggestions** by Paula M. Bousquet, Judith Fitzsimmons; ISBN: 1573245569; http://www.amazon.com/exec/obidos/ASIN/1573245569/icongroupinterna

- **Aromatherapy to Heal & Tend the Body** by Robert Tisserand (1988); ISBN: 0941524426;
  http://www.amazon.com/exec/obidos/ASIN/0941524426/icongroupinterna

- **Aromatherapy Treatments: A Practical Way to Health and Enjoyment for Body, Mind and Spirit** by Marion Wayman (2003); ISBN: 9654941376;
  http://www.amazon.com/exec/obidos/ASIN/9654941376/icongroupinterna

- **AROMATHERAPY USING ESSENTIAL OILS** by RYMAN; ISBN: 0752900471;
  http://www.amazon.com/exec/obidos/ASIN/0752900471/icongroupinterna

- **Aromatherapy Workbook** by Marcel Lavabre, Marcel Levabre; ISBN: 0892816449;
  http://www.amazon.com/exec/obidos/ASIN/0892816449/icongroupinterna

- **Aromatherapy Workshop** by Nicole Perez (2000); ISBN: 1861262566;
  http://www.amazon.com/exec/obidos/ASIN/1861262566/icongroupinterna

- **Aromatherapy: A Complete Guide to the Healing Art** by Kathy Keville, et al (1995); ISBN: 0895946920;
  http://www.amazon.com/exec/obidos/ASIN/0895946920/icongroupinterna

- **Aromatherapy: a Definitive Guide to Essential Oils** by Lisa Chidell; ISBN: 034056332X;
  http://www.amazon.com/exec/obidos/ASIN/034056332X/icongroupinterna

- **Aromatherapy: A Guide for Home Use** by Christine Westwood (1991); ISBN: 0951772309;
  http://www.amazon.com/exec/obidos/ASIN/0951772309/icongroupinterna

- **Aromatherapy: A Holistic Guide: Balance the Body and Soul With Essential Oils** by Ann Berwick; ISBN: 0875420338;
  http://www.amazon.com/exec/obidos/ASIN/0875420338/icongroupinterna

- **Aromatherapy: A Lifetime Guide to Healing With Essential Oils** by Valerie Cooksley; ISBN: 0133494322;
  http://www.amazon.com/exec/obidos/ASIN/0133494322/icongroupinterna

- **Aromatherapy: A Personal Journey Through Your Senses** by Patricia Betty (1994); ISBN: 0964120542;
  http://www.amazon.com/exec/obidos/ASIN/0964120542/icongroupinterna

- **Aromatherapy: A Practical Guide** by Marion Wayman (1999); ISBN: 9654940523;
  http://www.amazon.com/exec/obidos/ASIN/9654940523/icongroupinterna

- **Aromatherapy: A Practical Introduction** by Sandra White (1999); ISBN: 157145215X;
  http://www.amazon.com/exec/obidos/ASIN/157145215X/icongroupinterna

- **Aromatherapy: A Step-By-Step Guide ("In a Nutshell" Series)** by Sheila Lavery, et al; ISBN: 1862040125;
  http://www.amazon.com/exec/obidos/ASIN/1862040125/icongroupinterna

- **Aromatherapy: An Illustrated Guide** by Clare Walters; ISBN: 1862041660;
  http://www.amazon.com/exec/obidos/ASIN/1862041660/icongroupinterna

- **Aromatherapy: an Introduction to Alternative Health Care** by Sylvia Nichols (1996); ISBN: 1874445052;
  http://www.amazon.com/exec/obidos/ASIN/1874445052/icongroupinterna

- **Aromatherapy: An Introductory Guide to Professional and Home Use** by Gill Martin (1997); ISBN: 0091812763;
  http://www.amazon.com/exec/obidos/ASIN/0091812763/icongroupinterna

- **Aromatherapy: Essential Oils and How to Use Them** by Charla Devereux (2002); ISBN: 0804834709;
  http://www.amazon.com/exec/obidos/ASIN/0804834709/icongroupinterna

- **Aromatherapy: Essential Oils for Vibrant Health and Beauty** by Roberta Wison, et al (2002); ISBN: 1583331301;
  http://www.amazon.com/exec/obidos/ASIN/1583331301/icongroupinterna

- **Aromatherapy: Essential Oils in Colour** by Rosemary Caddy (1997); ISBN: 1899308148;
  http://www.amazon.com/exec/obidos/ASIN/1899308148/icongroupinterna

- **Aromatherapy: Fact and Fiction** by Maria Lis Ph.D. Balchin, Charla Devereux; ISBN: 0750647604;
  http://www.amazon.com/exec/obidos/ASIN/0750647604/icongroupinterna

- **Aromatherapy: For Health and Harmony (Health and Well - Being)** by Mark Evans, Don Last (Photographer) (2000); ISBN: 1842151754;
  http://www.amazon.com/exec/obidos/ASIN/1842151754/icongroupinterna

- **Aromatherapy: For Health, Well-Being and Relaxation** by Joanne Rippin; ISBN: 1859675565;
  http://www.amazon.com/exec/obidos/ASIN/1859675565/icongroupinterna

- **Aromatherapy: For Relaxation, Beauty and Good Health** by Glenda Taylor; ISBN: 0688174906;
  http://www.amazon.com/exec/obidos/ASIN/0688174906/icongroupinterna

- **Aromatherapy: Health and Beauty Care with Massage and Essentia Oils** by Micheline Arcier; ISBN: 0600568210;
  http://www.amazon.com/exec/obidos/ASIN/0600568210/icongroupinterna

- **Aromatherapy: Massage With Essential Oils (Health Essentials Series)** by Christine Wildwood; ISBN: 1862040974;
  http://www.amazon.com/exec/obidos/ASIN/1862040974/icongroupinterna

- **Aromatherapy: Principles & Practice** by Carol Horrigan, Nicole Perez; ISBN: 0750638079;
  http://www.amazon.com/exec/obidos/ASIN/0750638079/icongroupinterna

- **Aromatherapy: Recipes for Beauty, Health, and Well-Being** by Victoria H. Edwards (2003); ISBN: 158017891X;
  http://www.amazon.com/exec/obidos/ASIN/158017891X/icongroupinterna

- **Aromatherapy: Recipes for Your Oil Burner** by Judy Chapman, Katie Mitchell (1998); ISBN: 0732259142;
  http://www.amazon.com/exec/obidos/ASIN/0732259142/icongroupinterna

- **Aromatherapy: Revitalizing Mind & Body With Natural Fragrances** by Jo Richardson (Editor); ISBN: 1571455671;
  http://www.amazon.com/exec/obidos/ASIN/1571455671/icongroupinterna

- **Aromatherapy: Scentual** by Judith White, K. R. Day; ISBN: 0517419807;
  http://www.amazon.com/exec/obidos/ASIN/0517419807/icongroupinterna

- **Aromatherapy: Simply for You** by Marion Del Gaudio Mak (1999); ISBN: 1899308105;
  http://www.amazon.com/exec/obidos/ASIN/1899308105/icongroupinterna

- **Aromatherapy: Soothing Remedies to Restore, Rejuvenate and Heal** by Valerie Gennari, Rn Cooksley; ISBN: 073520361X;
  http://www.amazon.com/exec/obidos/ASIN/073520361X/icongroupinterna

- **Aromatherapy: Teach Yourself (Teach Yourself Books (Lincolnwood, Ill.).)** by Denise Whichello Brown (1996); ISBN: 0844231029; http://www.amazon.com/exec/obidos/ASIN/0844231029/icongroupinterna

- **Aromatherapy: The A-Z Guide to Healing With Essential Oils (The Essential Healing Arts Series)** by Shelagh Ryan Masline, Barbara Close; ISBN: 0440222567; http://www.amazon.com/exec/obidos/ASIN/0440222567/icongroupinterna

- **Aromatherapy: The Complete Guide to Plant and Flower Essences for Health and Beauty** by Daniele Ryman; ISBN: 0553371665; http://www.amazon.com/exec/obidos/ASIN/0553371665/icongroupinterna

- **Aromatherapy: The Encyclopedia of Plants and Oils and How They Help You** by Daniele Ryman; ISBN: 0749910801; http://www.amazon.com/exec/obidos/ASIN/0749910801/icongroupinterna

- **Aromatherapy: The Essential Blending Guide** by Rosemary Caddy (2000); ISBN: 1899308245; http://www.amazon.com/exec/obidos/ASIN/1899308245/icongroupinterna

- **Aromatherapy: The Pregnancy Book** by Jennie Supper (1999); ISBN: 1899308202; http://www.amazon.com/exec/obidos/ASIN/1899308202/icongroupinterna

- **Aromatherapy: Therapy Basics: Answers (Therapy Basics)** by Helen McGuinness; ISBN: 034070151X; http://www.amazon.com/exec/obidos/ASIN/034070151X/icongroupinterna

- **Aromatic Aromatherapy for the Home: Pot Pourris, Oils and Scented Decorations to Enhance Your Home** by Angela Flanders; ISBN: 0753702851; http://www.amazon.com/exec/obidos/ASIN/0753702851/icongroupinterna

- **Art of Aromatherapy** by Random House Value Publishing (2000); ISBN: 0517203235; http://www.amazon.com/exec/obidos/ASIN/0517203235/icongroupinterna

- **Astrological Aromatherapy** by Patricia Davis, Diane Melanie (Illustrator) (2002); ISBN: 0852073569; http://www.amazon.com/exec/obidos/ASIN/0852073569/icongroupinterna

- **Ayurveda & Aromatherapy, Earth Guide** by Dr. Light Miller, et al (1995); ISBN: 0914955209; http://www.amazon.com/exec/obidos/ASIN/0914955209/icongroupinterna

- **Beautiful Skin With Aromatherapy** by June Thornton (1998); ISBN: 0670882291; http://www.amazon.com/exec/obidos/ASIN/0670882291/icongroupinterna

- **Becoming an Aromatherapist: The Complete Guide to Training and Working in Aromatherapy** by Rhiannon Harris (2001); ISBN: 1857036824; http://www.amazon.com/exec/obidos/ASIN/1857036824/icongroupinterna

- **Bloomsbury Encyclopedia of Aromatherapy** by Chrissie Wildwood; ISBN: 0747550557; http://www.amazon.com/exec/obidos/ASIN/0747550557/icongroupinterna

- **Carrier Oils for Aromatherapy & Massage** by Leonard Price; ISBN: 1874353026; http://www.amazon.com/exec/obidos/ASIN/1874353026/icongroupinterna

- **Clinical Aromatherapy for Pregnancy and Childbirth** by Denise Tiran (Editor), Sue Mack (Editor) (2000); ISBN: 044306427X; http://www.amazon.com/exec/obidos/ASIN/044306427X/icongroupinterna

- **Clinical Aromatherapy: Essential Oils in Practice** by Jane Buckle (2003); ISBN: 0443072361;
  http://www.amazon.com/exec/obidos/ASIN/0443072361/icongroupinterna

- **Comforting Scents: A Personal Aromatherapy Journal** by Valerie Cooksley, Doug Corcoran (Editor); ISBN: 0735200025;
  http://www.amazon.com/exec/obidos/ASIN/0735200025/icongroupinterna

- **Common Scents: A Practical Guide to Aromatherapy** by Lorrie Hargis; ISBN: 1580540708;
  http://www.amazon.com/exec/obidos/ASIN/1580540708/icongroupinterna

- **Complete Aromatherapy Gift Set/Includes 8 Pure Essential Oils, Eyedropper and Complete Aromatherapy Handbook** by Susanne Fischer-Rizzi; ISBN: 0806956879;
  http://www.amazon.com/exec/obidos/ASIN/0806956879/icongroupinterna

- **Complete Aromatherapy Handbook: Essential Oils for Radiant Health** by Susanne Fischer-Rizzi, et al (1991); ISBN: 0806982225;
  http://www.amazon.com/exec/obidos/ASIN/0806982225/icongroupinterna

- **Complete Aromatherapy Hdbk** by Storey Publishing (1997); ISBN: 0676571980;
  http://www.amazon.com/exec/obidos/ASIN/0676571980/icongroupinterna

- **Complete Aromatherapy Massage Gift Pack (The Complete Book)**; ISBN: 0751325856;
  http://www.amazon.com/exec/obidos/ASIN/0751325856/icongroupinterna

- **Complete Guide to Massage, Aromatherapy & Yoga (Practical Handbook Series)** by Carole McGilvery, et al; ISBN: 0754800237;
  http://www.amazon.com/exec/obidos/ASIN/0754800237/icongroupinterna

- **Create Your Own Aromatherapy Perfumes: Enchanting Blends for Body and Home** by Chrissie Wildwood (1999); ISBN: 0749919647;
  http://www.amazon.com/exec/obidos/ASIN/0749919647/icongroupinterna

- **Creating Fairy Garden Fragrances (The Spirit of Aromatherapy)** by Linda K. Gannon (1998); ISBN: 1580170765;
  http://www.amazon.com/exec/obidos/ASIN/1580170765/icongroupinterna

- **Creative Aromatherapy** by Christine Wildwood; ISBN: 0722529201;
  http://www.amazon.com/exec/obidos/ASIN/0722529201/icongroupinterna

- **Culpeper Herbs & Aromatherapy** by Joannah Metcalfe; ISBN: 1860198066;
  http://www.amazon.com/exec/obidos/ASIN/1860198066/icongroupinterna

- **Daniele Ryman's Aromatherapy Bible** by Daniele Ryman; ISBN: 074992313X;
  http://www.amazon.com/exec/obidos/ASIN/074992313X/icongroupinterna

- **DK Living: Aromatherapy Massage (DK Living)** by Clare Maxwell-Hudson; ISBN: 0751307408;
  http://www.amazon.com/exec/obidos/ASIN/0751307408/icongroupinterna

- **Dk Living: Aromatherapy Massage (Special Version for Am** by None; ISBN: 075133345X;
  http://www.amazon.com/exec/obidos/ASIN/075133345X/icongroupinterna

- **Do-It-Yourself Natural Health: Acupressure, Herbal, & Aromatherapy** by John Sherman; ISBN: 0970941110;
  http://www.amazon.com/exec/obidos/ASIN/0970941110/icongroupinterna

- **Easy Steps to Aromatherapy** by Rosalind Widdowson (1995); ISBN: 1572150807;
  http://www.amazon.com/exec/obidos/ASIN/1572150807/icongroupinterna

- **Easy Steps to Aromatherapy** (1995); ISBN: 1856277429;
  http://www.amazon.com/exec/obidos/ASIN/1856277429/icongroupinterna

- **Egyptian Luxuries: Fragrance, Aromatherapy, and Cosmetics in Pharaonic Times** by Lise Manniche, Werner Forman; ISBN: 9774245350;
  http://www.amazon.com/exec/obidos/ASIN/9774245350/icongroupinterna

- **Enchanting Scents (Secrets of Aromatherapy)** by Monika Junemann, Monika Juenemann (1998); ISBN: 0941524361;
  http://www.amazon.com/exec/obidos/ASIN/0941524361/icongroupinterna

- **Encyclopedia of Aromatherapy** by Storey Publishing (1997); ISBN: 0676571107;
  http://www.amazon.com/exec/obidos/ASIN/0676571107/icongroupinterna

- **Encyclopedia of Aromatherapy** (1997); ISBN: 0752521578;
  http://www.amazon.com/exec/obidos/ASIN/0752521578/icongroupinterna

- **Encyclopedia of Aromatherapy** by Christine Wildwood; ISBN: 0892816384;
  http://www.amazon.com/exec/obidos/ASIN/0892816384/icongroupinterna

- **Encyclopedia of Essential Oils: The Complete Guide to the Use of Aromatic Oils in Aromatherapy, Herbalism, Health & Well-Being** by Julia Lawless (2002); ISBN: 0007145187;
  http://www.amazon.com/exec/obidos/ASIN/0007145187/icongroupinterna

- **Erotic Aromatherapy: Essential Oils for Lovers** by Chrissie Wildwood, George Dodd; ISBN: 0806907363;
  http://www.amazon.com/exec/obidos/ASIN/0806907363/icongroupinterna

- **Esencia De LA Aromaterapia/Essence of Aromatherapy** by Carolina Da Silva, et al (2000); ISBN: 1567182380;
  http://www.amazon.com/exec/obidos/ASIN/1567182380/icongroupinterna

- **Essence Of Aromatherapy**; ISBN: 0836252268;
  http://www.amazon.com/exec/obidos/ASIN/0836252268/icongroupinterna

- **Essence of Love : Fragrance, Aphrodisiacs, and Aromatherapy for Lovers** by Maggie Tisserand (Author) (1994); ISBN: 0062509144;
  http://www.amazon.com/exec/obidos/ASIN/0062509144/icongroupinterna

- **Essential Aromatherapy** by Storey Publishing (1997); ISBN: 0676571409;
  http://www.amazon.com/exec/obidos/ASIN/0676571409/icongroupinterna

- **Essential Aromatherapy** (1995); ISBN: 9994807870;
  http://www.amazon.com/exec/obidos/ASIN/9994807870/icongroupinterna

- **Essential Aromatherapy Book** by Carole Mcgilvery (Author); ISBN: 1859671373;
  http://www.amazon.com/exec/obidos/ASIN/1859671373/icongroupinterna

- **ESSENTIAL AROMATHERAPY TEXTBOOK**; ISBN: 0722529341;
  http://www.amazon.com/exec/obidos/ASIN/0722529341/icongroupinterna

- **Essential Aromatherapy: A Full-Color Guide to Using Essential Oils for Health Relaxation and Pleasure** by Carole McGilvery, Jimi Reed (Contributor); ISBN: 0831765062;
  http://www.amazon.com/exec/obidos/ASIN/0831765062/icongroupinterna

- **Essential Aromatherapy: A Pocket Guide to Essential Oils and Aromatherapy** by Susan E. Worwood, Valerie Ann Worwood (2003); ISBN: 1577312481;
  http://www.amazon.com/exec/obidos/ASIN/1577312481/icongroupinterna

- **Essential Chemistry for Safe Aromatherapy** by David Lowe, et al; ISBN: 0443064857;
  http://www.amazon.com/exec/obidos/ASIN/0443064857/icongroupinterna

- **Essential Energy: A Guide to Aromatherapy & Essential Oils** by Nikki Goldstein, et al;
  ISBN: 0446912093;
  http://www.amazon.com/exec/obidos/ASIN/0446912093/icongroupinterna

- **Everybody's Aromatherapy: A Comprehensive Guide for All Ages** by Helen Ranger;
  ISBN: 0624039447;
  http://www.amazon.com/exec/obidos/ASIN/0624039447/icongroupinterna

- **Everyday Aromatherapy Pack**; ISBN: 1860190162;
  http://www.amazon.com/exec/obidos/ASIN/1860190162/icongroupinterna

- **Facelift at Your Fingertips: An Aromatherapy Massage Program for Healthy Skin and a Younger Face** by Pierre Jean Cousin; ISBN: 1580172423;
  http://www.amazon.com/exec/obidos/ASIN/1580172423/icongroupinterna

- **Family Aromatherapy** by Joan Radford; ISBN: 0572024363;
  http://www.amazon.com/exec/obidos/ASIN/0572024363/icongroupinterna

- **Family Matters: Aromatherapy**; ISBN: 1850792658;
  http://www.amazon.com/exec/obidos/ASIN/1850792658/icongroupinterna

- **FAQs All About Aromatherapy** by Mindy Green; ISBN: 1583330321;
  http://www.amazon.com/exec/obidos/ASIN/1583330321/icongroupinterna

- **First Steps in Aromatherapy: A Simple and Straightforward Guide, Listing 58 Essential Oils** by Jane Dye (1996); ISBN: 0852072929;
  http://www.amazon.com/exec/obidos/ASIN/0852072929/icongroupinterna

- **Flower Power: Flower Remedies for Healing Body and Soul Through Herbalism, Homeopathy, Aromatherapy, and Flower Essences (Henry Holt Reference Book)** by Anne McIntyre; ISBN: 0805042164;
  http://www.amazon.com/exec/obidos/ASIN/0805042164/icongroupinterna

- **Frankincense & Myrrh: Through the Ages and a Complete Guide to Their Use in Herbalism and Aromatherapy Today** by Wanda Sellar (Contributor), et al (1997); ISBN: 0852073062;
  http://www.amazon.com/exec/obidos/ASIN/0852073062/icongroupinterna

- **Gattefosse's Aromatherapy the First Book on Aromatherapy**; ISBN: 0685355926;
  http://www.amazon.com/exec/obidos/ASIN/0685355926/icongroupinterna

- **Gattefosse's Aromatherapy the First Book on Aromatherapy** by Rene-Maurice Gattefosse, Robert B. Tisserand (Editor) (1993); ISBN: 0852072368;
  http://www.amazon.com/exec/obidos/ASIN/0852072368/icongroupinterna

- **GD: Ency Aromatherapy Massage**; ISBN: 721600003X;
  http://www.amazon.com/exec/obidos/ASIN/721600003X/icongroupinterna

- **GE: Aromatherapy**; ISBN: 7215967328;
  http://www.amazon.com/exec/obidos/ASIN/7215967328/icongroupinterna

- **Gentle Aromatherapy For Woman Decoder** by Dynamo House; ISBN: 1876100133;
  http://www.amazon.com/exec/obidos/ASIN/1876100133/icongroupinterna

- **Guide to Aromatherapy (The Brockhampton Library)**; ISBN: 1860192572;
  http://www.amazon.com/exec/obidos/ASIN/1860192572/icongroupinterna

- **Healing Spirit: Aromatherapy**; ISBN: 1840262281;
  http://www.amazon.com/exec/obidos/ASIN/1840262281/icongroupinterna

- **Healing With Aromatherapy** by Marlene Ericksen, Marlene Erickson; ISBN: 0658003828;
  http://www.amazon.com/exec/obidos/ASIN/0658003828/icongroupinterna

- **Healing With Aromatherapy: A Concise Guide to Using Essential Oils to Enhance Your Life (Essentials for Health & Harmony)** by Mark Evans, Southwater Publishing (2001); ISBN: 1842153803;
  http://www.amazon.com/exec/obidos/ASIN/1842153803/icongroupinterna

- **Health and Beauty Through Aromatherapy** by BLOSSOM KOCHHAR; ISBN: 8185944385;
  http://www.amazon.com/exec/obidos/ASIN/8185944385/icongroupinterna

- **Herbal Well-Being: Simple Recipes for Making Your Own Herbal Medicines, Aromatherapy Blends, and Herbal Body-Care Formulas** by Joyce A. Wardwell, et al (2002); ISBN: 1571458131;
  http://www.amazon.com/exec/obidos/ASIN/1571458131/icongroupinterna

- **Herbs & Aromatherapy for the Reproductive System: Men and Women (Jeanne Rose Earth Medicine Books)** by Jeanne Rose; ISBN: 188331917X;
  http://www.amazon.com/exec/obidos/ASIN/188331917X/icongroupinterna

- **Herbs and Aromatherapy** by Joannah Metcalfe (Author); ISBN: 1854710729;
  http://www.amazon.com/exec/obidos/ASIN/1854710729/icongroupinterna

- **Holistic Aromatherapy** by Christine Wildwood; ISBN: 0722528256;
  http://www.amazon.com/exec/obidos/ASIN/0722528256/icongroupinterna

- **Holistic Aromatherapy for Animals: A Comprehensive Guide to the Use of Essential Oils and Hydrosols With Animals** by Kristen Leigh Bell; ISBN: 1899171592;
  http://www.amazon.com/exec/obidos/ASIN/1899171592/icongroupinterna

- **Home Aromatherapy Kit - Including two Essential Oils, a Ceramic Ring and a Step-by-Step Guide to Essential Oils in the Home** by Julia Lawless; ISBN: 1856262057;
  http://www.amazon.com/exec/obidos/ASIN/1856262057/icongroupinterna

- **Home Aromatherapy: A Step-by-step Guide on Using Essential Oils at Home** by Julia Lawless; ISBN: 1856261743;
  http://www.amazon.com/exec/obidos/ASIN/1856261743/icongroupinterna

- **Home Aromatherapy: A Step-by-step Guide to Using Essential Oils in the Home** by Julia Lawless; ISBN: 1856261174;
  http://www.amazon.com/exec/obidos/ASIN/1856261174/icongroupinterna

- **Hydrosols: The Next Aromatherapy** by Suzanne Catty; ISBN: 0892819464;
  http://www.amazon.com/exec/obidos/ASIN/0892819464/icongroupinterna

- **Illustrated Elements of Aromatherapy** by Clare Walters (2003); ISBN: 0007150466;
  http://www.amazon.com/exec/obidos/ASIN/0007150466/icongroupinterna

- **Indulge Yourself with Aromatherapy** by M. Lou Luchsinger; ISBN: 0806927631;
  http://www.amazon.com/exec/obidos/ASIN/0806927631/icongroupinterna

- **Instant Aromatherapy** by Miriam Zellnik, Miriam Zellnik (2003); ISBN: 1931686750;
  http://www.amazon.com/exec/obidos/ASIN/1931686750/icongroupinterna

- **Instant Aromatherapy 8c Display**; ISBN: 1931686769;
  http://www.amazon.com/exec/obidos/ASIN/1931686769/icongroupinterna

- **Joy of Aromatherapy: Sensual Remedies for Everyday Ailments** by Cathy Hopkins; ISBN: 0207168717;
http://www.amazon.com/exec/obidos/ASIN/0207168717/icongroupinterna

- **Like Chocolate for Women: Indulge and Recharge with Everyday Aromatherapy** by Kim Morrison, et al (2002); ISBN: 1877178861;
http://www.amazon.com/exec/obidos/ASIN/1877178861/icongroupinterna

- **Liquid Sunshine: Vegetable Oils for Aromatherapy** by Jan Kusmirek (2003); ISBN: 0954329503;
http://www.amazon.com/exec/obidos/ASIN/0954329503/icongroupinterna

- **Magical Aromatherapy: The Power of Scent (Llewellyn's New Age Series)** by Scott Cunningham, Robert Tisserand; ISBN: 0875421296;
http://www.amazon.com/exec/obidos/ASIN/0875421296/icongroupinterna

- **Making Aromatherapy Creams and Lotions: 101 Natural Formulas to Revitalize & Nourish Your Skin** by Donna Maria, et al; ISBN: 1580172415;
http://www.amazon.com/exec/obidos/ASIN/1580172415/icongroupinterna

- **Making Herbal Dream Pillows : Secret Blends for Pleasant Dreams (The Spirit of Aromatherapy)** by Jim Long (1998); ISBN: 1580170757;
http://www.amazon.com/exec/obidos/ASIN/1580170757/icongroupinterna

- **Marguerite Maury's Guide to Aromatherapy: The Secret of Life and Youth** by Marguerite Maury, Danielle Ryman (1989); ISBN: 0852071639;
http://www.amazon.com/exec/obidos/ASIN/0852071639/icongroupinterna

- **Massage & Aromatherapy: A Practical Approach** by Lyn Goldberg (2001); ISBN: 0748758755;
http://www.amazon.com/exec/obidos/ASIN/0748758755/icongroupinterna

- **Massage and Aromatherapy: A Guide for Health Professionals** by A. Vickers (1996); ISBN: 0748740295;
http://www.amazon.com/exec/obidos/ASIN/0748740295/icongroupinterna

- **Massage and Aromatherapy: A Practical Approach for Nvq Level 3** by Lyn Goldberg (1999); ISBN: 0748720812;
http://www.amazon.com/exec/obidos/ASIN/0748720812/icongroupinterna

- **Medical Aromatherapy: Healing with Essential Oils** by Kurt Schnaubelt; ISBN: 1883319692;
http://www.amazon.com/exec/obidos/ASIN/1883319692/icongroupinterna

- **Meditations & Rituals Using Aromatherapy Oils** by Gil Farrer-Halls, Gill Farrer-Halls (2001); ISBN: 080692652X;
http://www.amazon.com/exec/obidos/ASIN/080692652X/icongroupinterna

- **More Aromatherapy Recipes from Around the World** by Judy Chapman, Katie Mitchell (2001); ISBN: 0732271355;
http://www.amazon.com/exec/obidos/ASIN/0732271355/icongroupinterna

- **Natural Bodycare: Creating Aromatherapy Cosmetics for Health & Beauty** by Julia Meadow (Photographer), et al; ISBN: 0806942452;
http://www.amazon.com/exec/obidos/ASIN/0806942452/icongroupinterna

- **Natural Healing With Aromatherapy** by Prentice-Hall, Ph Editorial (1996); ISBN: 013258963X;
http://www.amazon.com/exec/obidos/ASIN/013258963X/icongroupinterna

- **Natural Healing With Aromatherapy (Healthful Alternatives Series)** by Gisela Bulla; ISBN: 0806942215;
  http://www.amazon.com/exec/obidos/ASIN/0806942215/icongroupinterna

- **Natural Perfumes: Simple Aromatherapy Recipes** by Mindy Green (1999); ISBN: 1883010624;
  http://www.amazon.com/exec/obidos/ASIN/1883010624/icongroupinterna

- **Nature's Cures: From Acupressure & Aromatherapy to Walking & Yoga, the Ultimate Guide to the Best Scientifically Proven, Drug_Free Healing Methods** by Michael Castleman; ISBN: 0875963013;
  http://www.amazon.com/exec/obidos/ASIN/0875963013/icongroupinterna

- **New Choices in Natural Healing for Women: From Aromatherapy and Herbs to Massage and Vitamin Therapy--Drug-Free Remedies from the World of Alternative Medicine** by Barbara Loecher, et al; ISBN: 0875963870;
  http://www.amazon.com/exec/obidos/ASIN/0875963870/icongroupinterna

- **New Perspectives: Aromatherapy** by Christine Wildwood; ISBN: 1862046301;
  http://www.amazon.com/exec/obidos/ASIN/1862046301/icongroupinterna

- **Opportunity Profile: The Aromatherapy Consumer [DOWNLOAD: PDF]** by Natural Marketing Institute (Author); ISBN: B00005TYUM;
  http://www.amazon.com/exec/obidos/ASIN/B00005TYUM/icongroupinterna

- **Phyto-Aromatherapy in Clinical Practice** by Gabriel Mojay (Editor) (2003); ISBN: 0750640014;
  http://www.amazon.com/exec/obidos/ASIN/0750640014/icongroupinterna

- **Pocket Guide to Aromatherapy (The Crossing Press Pocket Series)** by Kathy Keville (1996); ISBN: 089594815X;
  http://www.amazon.com/exec/obidos/ASIN/089594815X/icongroupinterna

- **Portraits in Oils: The Personality of Aromatherapy Oils and Their Link With Human Temperaments** by Philippe Mailhebiau, et al (1996); ISBN: 0852072376;
  http://www.amazon.com/exec/obidos/ASIN/0852072376/icongroupinterna

- **Practical Aromatherapy** by Shirley Price; ISBN: 0722539061;
  http://www.amazon.com/exec/obidos/ASIN/0722539061/icongroupinterna

- **Practical Aromatherapy**; ISBN: 0752519336;
  http://www.amazon.com/exec/obidos/ASIN/0752519336/icongroupinterna

- **Practical Aromatherapy** (2000); ISBN: 0752534246;
  http://www.amazon.com/exec/obidos/ASIN/0752534246/icongroupinterna

- **Practical Aromatherapy** by Penny Rich (Author); ISBN: 1858137713;
  http://www.amazon.com/exec/obidos/ASIN/1858137713/icongroupinterna

- **Practical Aromatherapy** by Deborah Nixon (1996); ISBN: 1863024174;
  http://www.amazon.com/exec/obidos/ASIN/1863024174/icongroupinterna

- **Practical Aromatherapy For Home And Garden Decoder** by Dynamo House; ISBN: 1876100257;
  http://www.amazon.com/exec/obidos/ASIN/1876100257/icongroupinterna

- **Practical Aromatherapy Kit** by Deborah Nixon (1996); ISBN: 1863025162;
  http://www.amazon.com/exec/obidos/ASIN/1863025162/icongroupinterna

- **Practical Aromatherapy: The Complete Beginner's Guide to Choosing, Massaging, and Relaxing With Essential Oils** by Penny Rich (1994); ISBN: 0788161954;
http://www.amazon.com/exec/obidos/ASIN/0788161954/icongroupinterna

- **Practical Aromatherapy: the Complete Beginner's Guide (Black & White Paperbacks)** by Penny Rich; ISBN: 0752514296;
http://www.amazon.com/exec/obidos/ASIN/0752514296/icongroupinterna

- **Practical Aromatherapy: the Complete Beginners Guide to Choosing, Massaging and Relaxing with Essential Oils** by Penny Rich; ISBN: 1854873156;
http://www.amazon.com/exec/obidos/ASIN/1854873156/icongroupinterna

- **Practical Aromatherapy: Understanding and Using Essential Oils to Heal the Mind and Body** by Robyn M. Feller; ISBN: 0425155765;
http://www.amazon.com/exec/obidos/ASIN/0425155765/icongroupinterna

- **Practical Art of Aromatherapy** by Random House Value Publishing (2000); ISBN: 0517203251;
http://www.amazon.com/exec/obidos/ASIN/0517203251/icongroupinterna

- **Practical Art of Aromatherapy: Create Your Own Personalized Beauty Treatments and Natural Remedies** by Deborah Nixon (1996); ISBN: 0517142392;
http://www.amazon.com/exec/obidos/ASIN/0517142392/icongroupinterna

- **Practice of Aromatherapy: Holistic Health and the Essential Oils of Flowers and Herbs** by Jean Valnet, Robert Tisserand (Photographer); ISBN: 0892810262;
http://www.amazon.com/exec/obidos/ASIN/0892810262/icongroupinterna

- **Sacred Luxuries: Fragrance, Aromatherapy, and Cosmetics in Ancient Egypt** by Lise Manniche, Werner Forman (Photographer) (1999); ISBN: 0801437202;
http://www.amazon.com/exec/obidos/ASIN/0801437202/icongroupinterna

- **Salonovations' Guide to Aromatherapy** by Shelley Hess, Marlene Pratt (Editor); ISBN: 1562533134;
http://www.amazon.com/exec/obidos/ASIN/1562533134/icongroupinterna

- **Scent Sense: An Essential Guide to Aromatherapy (Cosmic Kits)** by Janet Denhard, et al; ISBN: 1901881563;
http://www.amazon.com/exec/obidos/ASIN/1901881563/icongroupinterna

- **Scents & Scentuality: Essential Oils & Aromatherapy for Romance, Love, and Sex** by Valerie Ann Worwood (1998); ISBN: 1577310756;
http://www.amazon.com/exec/obidos/ASIN/1577310756/icongroupinterna

- **Scentual Touch: A Personal Guide to Aromatherapy** by Judith Jackson, Richard Ely; ISBN: 0030067634;
http://www.amazon.com/exec/obidos/ASIN/0030067634/icongroupinterna

- **Seasons of Aromatherapy: Hundreds of Restorative Recipes and Sensory Suggestions** by Judith Fitzsimmons, et al (1999); ISBN: 157324144X;
http://www.amazon.com/exec/obidos/ASIN/157324144X/icongroupinterna

- **Secrets of Aromatherapy (Natural Care)** by Jennie Harding; ISBN: 0751312045;
http://www.amazon.com/exec/obidos/ASIN/0751312045/icongroupinterna

- **Sensual Aromatherapy**; ISBN: 7215971589;
http://www.amazon.com/exec/obidos/ASIN/7215971589/icongroupinterna

- **Sensual Aromatherapy Essential Oils For** by Chrissie Wildwood (Author); ISBN: 0747210632;
  http://www.amazon.com/exec/obidos/ASIN/0747210632/icongroupinterna

- **Setting the Mood With Aromatherapy** by Carly Wall, Joanna Roy (Illustrator) (1998); ISBN: 0806998717;
  http://www.amazon.com/exec/obidos/ASIN/0806998717/icongroupinterna

- **Soft Tissue Injuries: Management and Prevention Through Aromatherapy** by Maureen Farrell, Lesley Thompson; ISBN: 0750641649;
  http://www.amazon.com/exec/obidos/ASIN/0750641649/icongroupinterna

- **Step by Step Aromatherapy** by Renee Tanner; ISBN: 0951620320;
  http://www.amazon.com/exec/obidos/ASIN/0951620320/icongroupinterna

- **Stressbusting Book of Massage, Aromatherapy & Yoga: A Step-By-Step Guide to Spiritual and Physical Well-Being** by Carole McGilvery, et al (2002); ISBN: 1842155652;
  http://www.amazon.com/exec/obidos/ASIN/1842155652/icongroupinterna

- **Sublte Aromatherapy** by Patricia Davis (2000); ISBN: 0846442957;
  http://www.amazon.com/exec/obidos/ASIN/0846442957/icongroupinterna

- **Subtle Aromatherapy** by Patricia Davis, Patiricia Davis (1995); ISBN: 0852072279;
  http://www.amazon.com/exec/obidos/ASIN/0852072279/icongroupinterna

- **The Alchemy of Health : Herbal Medicine and Herbal Aromatherapy** by Amira Amara Sravesh, Amira Amarah Sravesh; ISBN: 0966668804;
  http://www.amazon.com/exec/obidos/ASIN/0966668804/icongroupinterna

- **The Ancient and Healing Art of Aromatherapy** by Clare Hill; ISBN: 1569750947;
  http://www.amazon.com/exec/obidos/ASIN/1569750947/icongroupinterna

- **The Aromatherapy and Massage Book** by Christine Wildwood; ISBN: 0722529759;
  http://www.amazon.com/exec/obidos/ASIN/0722529759/icongroupinterna

- **The Aromatherapy Book: Applications & Inhalations** by Jeanne Rose, John Hulburd (Illustrator) (1992); ISBN: 1556430736;
  http://www.amazon.com/exec/obidos/ASIN/1556430736/icongroupinterna

- **The Aromatherapy Companion: Medicinal Uses, Ayurvedic Healing, Body Care Blends, Perfumes & Scents, Emotional Health & Well-Being** by Victoria H. Edwards (1999); ISBN: 1580171508;
  http://www.amazon.com/exec/obidos/ASIN/1580171508/icongroupinterna

- **The Aromatherapy Garden** by Julia Lawless, et al; ISBN: 1856263754;
  http://www.amazon.com/exec/obidos/ASIN/1856263754/icongroupinterna

- **The Aromatherapy Gift Set** by Julia Lawless (1996); ISBN: 0895778378;
  http://www.amazon.com/exec/obidos/ASIN/0895778378/icongroupinterna

- **The Aromatherapy Gift Set** by BHB International; ISBN: 1858336953;
  http://www.amazon.com/exec/obidos/ASIN/1858336953/icongroupinterna

- **The Aromatherapy Handbook: The Secret Healing Power of Essential Oils** by Daniele Ryman (1989); ISBN: 0852072155;
  http://www.amazon.com/exec/obidos/ASIN/0852072155/icongroupinterna

- **The Aromatherapy Kit** by Charla Devereux, Bernie Hephrun (Designer); ISBN: 0804819815;
  http://www.amazon.com/exec/obidos/ASIN/0804819815/icongroupinterna

- **The Aromatherapy Kitchen: Recipes for Health and Beauty Using Essential Oils** by Nicola Jenkins (2001); ISBN: 0855328886;
http://www.amazon.com/exec/obidos/ASIN/0855328886/icongroupinterna

- **The aromatherapy pocket book** by Kendra Grace; ISBN: 0964419807;
http://www.amazon.com/exec/obidos/ASIN/0964419807/icongroupinterna

- **The Aromatherapy Studio: A Step-by-step Introduction to Aromatherapy**; ISBN: 185152651X;
http://www.amazon.com/exec/obidos/ASIN/185152651X/icongroupinterna

- **The Aromatherapy Workbook: Understanding Essential Oils from Plant to Bottle** by Shirley Price (1994); ISBN: 0722526458;
http://www.amazon.com/exec/obidos/ASIN/0722526458/icongroupinterna

- **The Art of Aromatherapy** by Clare Hill; ISBN: 0600592421;
http://www.amazon.com/exec/obidos/ASIN/0600592421/icongroupinterna

- **The Art of Aromatherapy: A Guide to Using Essential Oils for Health and Relaxation** by Pamela Allardice; ISBN: 0517120674;
http://www.amazon.com/exec/obidos/ASIN/0517120674/icongroupinterna

- **The Art of Aromatherapy: The Healing and Beautifying Properties of the Essential Oils of Flowers and Herbs** by Robert B. Tisserand (1987); ISBN: 0892810017;
http://www.amazon.com/exec/obidos/ASIN/0892810017/icongroupinterna

- **The Art of Sensual Aromatherapy: A Lover's Guide to Using Aromatic Oils and Essences** by Nitya Lacroix, Sakina Bowhay (Contributor); ISBN: 0805041532;
http://www.amazon.com/exec/obidos/ASIN/0805041532/icongroupinterna

- **The Autonomic Nervous System and Aromatherapy** by Jennine Stromkins, Trent Stromkins (Illustrator); ISBN: 0968435602;
http://www.amazon.com/exec/obidos/ASIN/0968435602/icongroupinterna

- **The Book of Aromatherapy and Massage** by N. Lacroix; ISBN: 1840385154;
http://www.amazon.com/exec/obidos/ASIN/1840385154/icongroupinterna

- **The Book of Aromatherapy Blends: How to Use Essential Oils and Flower Remedies Creatively** by Christine Wildwood; ISBN: 0722534531;
http://www.amazon.com/exec/obidos/ASIN/0722534531/icongroupinterna

- **The Book of Massage and Aromatherapy** by Nitya Lacroix, Sharon Seager (2002); ISBN: 0754809870;
http://www.amazon.com/exec/obidos/ASIN/0754809870/icongroupinterna

- **The Book of Practical Aromatherapy** by William H. Lee, et al; ISBN: 0879835397;
http://www.amazon.com/exec/obidos/ASIN/0879835397/icongroupinterna

- **The Book of Touch & Aroma: Sensual Ways With Massage and Aromatherapy** by Cynthia Blanche, Time-Life Books (1999); ISBN: 0783552564;
http://www.amazon.com/exec/obidos/ASIN/0783552564/icongroupinterna

- **The Complete Book of Essential Oils and Aromatherapy** by Valerie Ann Worwood (1991); ISBN: 0931432820;
http://www.amazon.com/exec/obidos/ASIN/0931432820/icongroupinterna

- **The Complete Book of Family Aromatherapy** by Joan Radford (1994); ISBN: 0572016220;
http://www.amazon.com/exec/obidos/ASIN/0572016220/icongroupinterna

- **The Complete Guide to Aromatherapy (Practical Handbooks)** by Carole McGilvery, Jimi Reed (2001); ISBN: 0754807746;
  http://www.amazon.com/exec/obidos/ASIN/0754807746/icongroupinterna

- **The Complete Home Guide to Aromatherapy** by Erich Keller, Nancy Carleton (Editor); ISBN: 0915811367;
  http://www.amazon.com/exec/obidos/ASIN/0915811367/icongroupinterna

- **The Complete Massage and Aromatherapy Kit**; ISBN: 1859673287;
  http://www.amazon.com/exec/obidos/ASIN/1859673287/icongroupinterna

- **The Encyclopaedia of Aromatherapy** by Christine Wildwood (2001); ISBN: 1856278549;
  http://www.amazon.com/exec/obidos/ASIN/1856278549/icongroupinterna

- **The Encyclopaedia of Aromatherapy, Massage and Yoga: A Comprehensive, Practical Guide to Natural Health, Relaxation and Vitality** by Carole McGilvery, et al; ISBN: 1840389222;
  http://www.amazon.com/exec/obidos/ASIN/1840389222/icongroupinterna

- **The Encyclopedia of Aromatherapy, Massage & Yoga** by McGilvery, et al; ISBN: 1840385367;
  http://www.amazon.com/exec/obidos/ASIN/1840385367/icongroupinterna

- **The Encyclopedia of Aromatherapy, Massage and Yoga** by Carole McGilvery, et al; ISBN: 1901289222;
  http://www.amazon.com/exec/obidos/ASIN/1901289222/icongroupinterna

- **The Encyclopedia of Aromatherapy, Massage and Yoga: A Practical Guide to Natural Ways to Health, Relaxation and Vitality** by Carole McGilvery, et al (1996); ISBN: 0831727411;
  http://www.amazon.com/exec/obidos/ASIN/0831727411/icongroupinterna

- **The Encyclopedia of Essential Oils: The Complete Guide to the Use of Aromatics in Aromatherapy, Herbalism, Health and Well-Being** by Julia Lawless (1992); ISBN: 1852303115;
  http://www.amazon.com/exec/obidos/ASIN/1852303115/icongroupinterna

- **The Encyclopedia of Healing Plants: A Guide to Aromatherapy, Flower Essences and Herbal Remedies** by Chrissie Wildwood; ISBN: 0749917105;
  http://www.amazon.com/exec/obidos/ASIN/0749917105/icongroupinterna

- **The Essence of Aromatherapy** by Glenda Taylor; ISBN: 1841720429;
  http://www.amazon.com/exec/obidos/ASIN/1841720429/icongroupinterna

- **The Essence of Magic: Tarot, Ritual, and Aromatherapy** by Mary K. Greer (1997); ISBN: 0880797185;
  http://www.amazon.com/exec/obidos/ASIN/0880797185/icongroupinterna

- **The Essential Aromatherapy Kit: A Full-Color Guide to Using Essential Oils for Health, Relaxation and Pleasure (Special Book- Plus Kids Series)** by Carole McGilvery, et al; ISBN: 1859671519;
  http://www.amazon.com/exec/obidos/ASIN/1859671519/icongroupinterna

- **The Essential Aromatherapy: A Comprehensive Guide to Using Essential Oils for Health, Relaxation and Pleasure** by Carole McGilvery, et al; ISBN: 1840384069;
  http://www.amazon.com/exec/obidos/ASIN/1840384069/icongroupinterna

- **The Fragrant Art of Aromatherapy** by John Sinclair; ISBN: 1863024638;
  http://www.amazon.com/exec/obidos/ASIN/1863024638/icongroupinterna

- **The Fragrant Mind: Aromatherapy for Personality, Mind, Mood, and Emotion** by Valerie Ann Worwood (1996); ISBN: 1880032910;
  http://www.amazon.com/exec/obidos/ASIN/1880032910/icongroupinterna

- **The Fragrant Pharmacy: A Home and Health Care Guide to Aromatherapy and Essential Oils** by Valerie Worwood; ISBN: 0333484428;
  http://www.amazon.com/exec/obidos/ASIN/0333484428/icongroupinterna

- **The Fragrant Year: Seasonal Meditations With Aromatherapy Oils** by Jane Grayson, Claire Hedges (Illustrator); ISBN: 0722528639;
  http://www.amazon.com/exec/obidos/ASIN/0722528639/icongroupinterna

- **The Healing Aromatherapy Bath: Therapeutic Treatments Using Meditation, Visualization & Essential Oils** by Margo Valentine Lazzara (1999); ISBN: 1580171974;
  http://www.amazon.com/exec/obidos/ASIN/1580171974/icongroupinterna

- **The Healing Power of Aromatherapy: The Enlightened Person's Guide to the Physical, Emotional, and Spiritual Benefits of Essential Oils** by Hasnain Walji (1996); ISBN: 0761504419;
  http://www.amazon.com/exec/obidos/ASIN/0761504419/icongroupinterna

- **The Healing Touch: The Power of Massage, Aromatherapy, Shiatsu and Reflexology for Health and Well-Being** by Suzanne Franzen, et al (2001); ISBN: 1842154060;
  http://www.amazon.com/exec/obidos/ASIN/1842154060/icongroupinterna

- **The Herbal Body Book: Herbs & Aromatherapy for Healthy Skin and Hair** by Jeanne Rose (1994); ISBN: 1879687046;
  http://www.amazon.com/exec/obidos/ASIN/1879687046/icongroupinterna

- **The Home Spa Aromatherapy Massage Set** by Bramley; ISBN: 1858337968;
  http://www.amazon.com/exec/obidos/ASIN/1858337968/icongroupinterna

- **The Illustrated Encyclopedia of Essential Oils: The Complete Guide to the Use of Oils in Aromatherapy and Herbalism** by Julia Lawless (1995); ISBN: 1852307218;
  http://www.amazon.com/exec/obidos/ASIN/1852307218/icongroupinterna

- **The Joy of Aromatherapy**; ISBN: 000637946X;
  http://www.amazon.com/exec/obidos/ASIN/000637946X/icongroupinterna

- **The Little Baby Massage Book: Complete With Acupressure and Aromatherapy Hands-On Massage Instruction to Give the Gift of Love and Touch to Your Baby** by Linda Ellen Larson, Stacie Sheridan (Illustrator) (2000); ISBN: 1587210010;
  http://www.amazon.com/exec/obidos/ASIN/1587210010/icongroupinterna

- **The Little Giant Encyclopaedia of Aromatherapy** by David Schiller, Carol Schiller; ISBN: 8170306906;
  http://www.amazon.com/exec/obidos/ASIN/8170306906/icongroupinterna

- **The Little Giant Encyclopedia of Aromatherapy** by David Schiller, Carol Schiller (1999); ISBN: 0806920653;
  http://www.amazon.com/exec/obidos/ASIN/0806920653/icongroupinterna

- **The Magick of Aromatherapy: The Use of Scent for Healing Body, Mind, and Spirit** by Gwydion O'Hara; ISBN: 1567183484;
  http://www.amazon.com/exec/obidos/ASIN/1567183484/icongroupinterna

- **The Massage Manual: A Complete Guide to the Therapeutic Arts of Massage and Aromatherapy** by Mark Evans (2002); ISBN: 0754809986;
  http://www.amazon.com/exec/obidos/ASIN/0754809986/icongroupinterna

- **The Power of Holistic Aromatherapy** by Christine Stead; ISBN: 0713716754;
  http://www.amazon.com/exec/obidos/ASIN/0713716754/icongroupinterna

- **The Practice of Aromatherapy** by Jean Valnet (1990); ISBN: 0846442736;
  http://www.amazon.com/exec/obidos/ASIN/0846442736/icongroupinterna

- **The Practice of Aromatherapy: A Classic Compendium of Plant Medicines and Their Healing Properties** by Jean Valnet, Robert Tisserand (Editor) (1990); ISBN: 0892813989;
  http://www.amazon.com/exec/obidos/ASIN/0892813989/icongroupinterna

- **The Soothing Touch of Partner Massage and Aromatherapy** by Brian Green, Royston Scott-Green (1995); ISBN: 0572019696;
  http://www.amazon.com/exec/obidos/ASIN/0572019696/icongroupinterna

- **The Ultimate Aromatherapy Pack** by Jo Richardson (Editor), et al (2002); ISBN: 184333027X;
  http://www.amazon.com/exec/obidos/ASIN/184333027X/icongroupinterna

- **The Ultimate Guide to Health from Nature: Vitamins, Minerals, Herbal Remedies, Bach Flower Remedies, and Aromatherapy Essential Oils** by Susan Holden, et al; ISBN: 9654941708;
  http://www.amazon.com/exec/obidos/ASIN/9654941708/icongroupinterna

- **The Very Essence: A Guide to Aromatherapy** by Lisa Burke (1996); ISBN: 0952842904;
  http://www.amazon.com/exec/obidos/ASIN/0952842904/icongroupinterna

- **The Very Essence: Guide to Aromatherapy** by Lisa Burke (1998); ISBN: 0952842939;
  http://www.amazon.com/exec/obidos/ASIN/0952842939/icongroupinterna

- **The World of Aromatherapy: An Anthology of Aromatic History, Ideas, Concepts and Case Histories** by Jeanne Rose (Editor), et al (1996); ISBN: 1883319498;
  http://www.amazon.com/exec/obidos/ASIN/1883319498/icongroupinterna

- **Thorsons Principles of Aromatherapy** by Cathy Hopkins; ISBN: 0722532636;
  http://www.amazon.com/exec/obidos/ASIN/0722532636/icongroupinterna

- **Traditional Aromatherapy (Traditional Series)** (1996); ISBN: 0752517325;
  http://www.amazon.com/exec/obidos/ASIN/0752517325/icongroupinterna

- **Ulla-Maija Grace's Aromatherapy for Practitioners** by Ulla-Maija Grace (1996); ISBN: 0852072937;
  http://www.amazon.com/exec/obidos/ASIN/0852072937/icongroupinterna

- **Veterinary Aromatherapy** by Nelly Grosjean (1994); ISBN: 0852072740;
  http://www.amazon.com/exec/obidos/ASIN/0852072740/icongroupinterna

- **Vibrational Healing: Revealing the Essence of Nature Through Aromatherapy's Use of Essential Oils** by Deborah Eidson; ISBN: 1583940316;
  http://www.amazon.com/exec/obidos/ASIN/1583940316/icongroupinterna

The National Library of Medicine Book Index

The National Library of Medicine at the National Institutes of Health has a massive database of books published on healthcare and biomedicine. Go to the following Internet site, **http://locatorplus.gov/**, and then select "Search LOCATORplus." Once you are in the search area, simply type "aromatherapy" (or synonyms) into the search box, and select "books only." From there, results can be sorted by publication date, author, or relevance. The following was recently catalogued by the National Library of Medicine:[7]

- **Advanced aromatherapy: the science of essential oil therapy** Author: Schnaubelt, Kurt.; Year: 1998; Rochester, Vt.: Healing Arts Press, 1998; ISBN: 0892817437
  http://www.amazon.com/exec/obidos/ASIN/0892817437/icongroupinterna

- **Alternative medicine sourcebook: basic consumer health information about alternative and complementary medical practices: including acupuncture, chiropractic, herbal medicine, homeopathy, naturopathic medicine, mind-body interventions ayurveda, and other non-westrern medical traditions: along with facts about such specific therapies as massage therapy, aromatherapy, qigong, hypnosis, prayer, dance, and art therapies, a glossary, and resources for further information** Author: Matthews, Dawn D.; Year: 1992; Detroit, MI: Omnigraphics, c2002; ISBN: 0780806050
  http://www.amazon.com/exec/obidos/ASIN/0780806050/icongroupinterna

- **Alternative medicine sourcebook: basic consumer health information about alternatives to conventional medicine, including acupressure, acupuncture, aromatherapy, ayurveda, bioelectromagnetics, environmental medicine, essence therapy, food and nutrition therapy, herbal therapy, homeopathy, imaging, massage, naturopathy, reflexology, relaxation and meditation, sound therapy, vitamin and mineral therapy, and yoga, and more** Author: Cook, Allan R.; Year: 1977; Detroit, MI: Omnigraphics, c1999; ISBN: 0780802004
  http://www.amazon.com/exec/obidos/ASIN/0780802004/icongroupinterna

- **Aromatherapy: a definitive guide to essential oils** Author: Chidell, Lisa.; Year: 9999; Dunton Green, Sevenoaks, Kent: Headway, 1992; ISBN: 034056332X
  http://www.amazon.com/exec/obidos/ASIN/034056332X/icongroupinterna

- **Aromatherapy for common ailments.** Author: Shirley Price; Year: 1991

- **Aromatherapy for health professionals** Author: Price, Shirley.; Year: 1999; Edinburgh; New York: Churchill Livingstone, 1999; ISBN: 0443062102
  http://www.amazon.com/exec/obidos/ASIN/0443062102/icongroupinterna

- **Aromatherapy for health professionals** Author: Price, Shirley.; Year: 2002; Edinburgh; New York: Churchill Livingstone, 1995; ISBN: 0443049750
  http://www.amazon.com/exec/obidos/ASIN/0443049750/icongroupinterna

- **Aromatherapy for the beauty therapist.** Author: Worwood, Valerie Ann; Year: 1993; London, England: Thomson Learning, Hairdressing and Beauty Industry Authority, 2001; ISBN: 1861526636
  http://www.amazon.com/exec/obidos/ASIN/1861526636/icongroupinterna

- **Aromatherapy in midwifery practice** Author: Tiran, Denise.; Year: 2002; London; Philadelphia: Bailliere Tindall, c1996; ISBN: 070201978X
  http://www.amazon.com/exec/obidos/ASIN/070201978X/icongroupinterna

- **Clinical aromatherapy: essential oils in practice** Author: Buckle, Jane,; Year: 1996; Philadelphia, PA: Churchill Livingstone, c2003; ISBN: 0443072361

---

[7] In addition to LOCATORPlus, in collaboration with authors and publishers, the National Center for Biotechnology Information (NCBI) is currently adapting biomedical books for the Web. The books may be accessed in two ways: (1) by searching directly using any search term or phrase (in the same way as the bibliographic database PubMed), or (2) by following the links to PubMed abstracts. Each PubMed abstract has a "Books" button that displays a facsimile of the abstract in which some phrases are hypertext links. These phrases are also found in the books available at NCBI. Click on hyperlinked results in the list of books in which the phrase is found. Currently, the majority of the links are between the books and PubMed. In the future, more links will be created between the books and other types of information, such as gene and protein sequences and macromolecular structures. See **http://www.ncbi.nlm.nih.gov/entrez/query.fcgi?db=Books**.

http://www.amazon.com/exec/obidos/ASIN/0443072361/icongroupinterna

- **Clinical aromatherapy for pregnancy and childbirth** Author: Tiran, Denise.; Year: 2000; Edinburgh; New York: Churchill Livingstone, 2000; ISBN: 044306427X
  http://www.amazon.com/exec/obidos/ASIN/044306427X/icongroupinterna

- **Clinical aromatherapy in nursing** Author: Buckle, Jane,; Year: 1999; San Diego, Calif.: Singular Pub. Group, c1997; ISBN: 1565938763

- **Complete aromatherapy handbook: essential oils for radiant health** Author: Fischer-Rizzi, Susanne.; Year: 2001; New York: Sterling Pub. Co., c1990; ISBN: 0806982225
  http://www.amazon.com/exec/obidos/ASIN/0806982225/icongroupinterna

- **Essential chemistry for safe aromatherapy** Author: Clarke, Sue,; Year: 1994; Edinburgh; New York: Churchill Livingstone, 2002; ISBN: 0443064857
  http://www.amazon.com/exec/obidos/ASIN/0443064857/icongroupinterna

- **Gattefossé's aromatherapy** Author: Gattefossé, René-Maurice,; Year: 2001; Saffron Walden: C.W. Daniel Co., 1993; ISBN: 0852072368
  http://www.amazon.com/exec/obidos/ASIN/0852072368/icongroupinterna

- **Hydrosols: the next aromatherapy** Author: Catty, Suzanne.; Year: 2000; Rochester, Vt.: Healing Arts Press, c2001; ISBN: 0892819464
  http://www.amazon.com/exec/obidos/ASIN/0892819464/icongroupinterna

- **Medical aromatherapy: healing with essential oils** Author: Schnaubelt, Kurt.; Year: 2003; Berkeley, Calif.: Frog, Ltd., c1999; ISBN: 1883319692
  http://www.amazon.com/exec/obidos/ASIN/1883319692/icongroupinterna

- **Sacred luxuries: fragrance, aromatherapy, and cosmetics in Ancient Egypt** Author: Manniche, Lise.; Year: 1998; Ithaca, N.Y.: Cornell University Press, 1999; ISBN: 0801437202
  http://www.amazon.com/exec/obidos/ASIN/0801437202/icongroupinterna

- **The aromatherapy book: applications & inhalations** Author: Rose, Jeanne.; Year: 2001; San Francisco: Herbal Studies Course, c1992; ISBN: 1556430736
  http://www.amazon.com/exec/obidos/ASIN/1556430736/icongroupinterna

- **The aromatherapy handbook: the secret healing power of essential oils** Author: Ryman, Danièle.; Year: 1996; London: Century Pub., 1984; ISBN: 071260328X
  http://www.amazon.com/exec/obidos/ASIN/071260328X/icongroupinterna

- **The art of aromatherapy: the healing and beautifying properties of the essential oils of flowers and herbs** Author: Tisserand, Robert.; Year: 2001; Rochester, Vt.: Healing Arts Press, c1977; ISBN: 0892810017
  http://www.amazon.com/exec/obidos/ASIN/0892810017/icongroupinterna

- **The art of aromatherapy.** Author: Tisserand, Robert.; Year: 1990; London: Daniel, c1977; ISBN: 085207140X
  http://www.amazon.com/exec/obidos/ASIN/085207140X/icongroupinterna

- **The complete book of essential oils and aromatherapy** Author: Worwood, Valerie Ann,; Year: 2001; San Rafael, Calif.: New World Library, c1991; ISBN: 0931432820
  http://www.amazon.com/exec/obidos/ASIN/0931432820/icongroupinterna

- **Ulla-Maija Grace's aromatherapy for practitioners** Author: Grace, Ulla-Maija.; Year: 1998; Saffron Walden, Essex, UK: C.W. Daniel Co., 1996; ISBN: 0852072937
  http://www.amazon.com/exec/obidos/ASIN/0852072937/icongroupinterna

Chapters on Aromatherapy

In order to find chapters that specifically relate to aromatherapy, an excellent source of abstracts is the Combined Health Information Database. You will need to limit your search to book chapters and aromatherapy using the "Detailed Search" option. Go to the following hyperlink: **http://chid.nih.gov/detail/detail.html** To find book chapters, use the drop boxes at the bottom of the search page where "You may refine your search by." Select the dates and language you prefer, and the format option "Book Chapter." Type "aromatherapy" (or synonyms) into the "For these words:" box. The following is a typical result when searching for book chapters on aromatherapy:

- **Alternative Medicine**

  Source: in Stein, S.H. and Rood, R.P. Inflammatory Bowel Disease: A Guide for Patients and Their Families. 2nd ed. Philadelphia, PA: Lippincott-Raven Publishers. 1999. p. 175-193.

  Contact: Available from Crohn's and Colitis Foundation of America. 386 Park Avenue South, 17th Floor, New York, NY 10016-8804. (800) 932-2423. Fax (212) 779-4098. E-mail: orders@ccfa.org. Website: www.ccfa.org. PRICE: $17.00 for members; $22.00 for nonmembers; plus shipping and handling. ISBN: 0397517718.

  Summary: While there is continued progress in treating inflammatory bowel disease (IBD), more people are turning to alternative modalities to try to relieve their symptoms. This chapter on alternative medicine in IBD is from a text written specifically for people with inflammatory bowel disease (IBD), which is the collective term for ulcerative colitis and Crohn's disease. Ulcerative colitis is an inflammatory disease of the large intestine (the colon), that is characterized by inflammation and ulceration of its inner lining. By contrast, Crohn's disease can affect any area of the gastrointestinal tract, including the small intestine. The author stresses that the biggest single problem with alternative medicine is the lack of responsible, scientifically based information on the safety, potential effects, and long term effects of alternative modalities. The author uses the term integrative medicine to refer to the integration of allopathic medicine and alternative therapies. The author stresses the benefits of allopathic medicine and cautions against using any physician or practitioner who suggests that Western medical care not be used or who will not work with or coordinate activities with a primary care physician or gastroenterologist. Topics covered include insurance coverage for alternative medicine for IBD, medical training, herbal remedies, manipulation therapy, massage therapy, acupuncture and traditional Chinese medicine, music and music beds, homeopathy, **aromatherapy,** psychoneuroimmunology, and prayer. The author concludes by reiterating the importance of combining traditional and alternative approaches to the treatment of IBD.

Directories

In addition to the references and resources discussed earlier in this chapter, a number of directories relating to aromatherapy have been published that consolidate information across various sources. The Combined Health Information Database lists the following, which you may wish to consult in your local medical library:[8]

---

[8] You will need to limit your search to "Directory" and "aromatherapy" using the "Detailed Search" option. Go directly to the following hyperlink: **http://chid.nih.gov/detail/detail.html**. To find directories, use the drop boxes at

- **Directory of Schools for Alternative and Complementary Health Care**

Source: Phoenix, AZ: Oryx Press. 1998. 250 p.

Contact: Oryx Press. PO Box 33889, Phoenix, AZ 85067-3889. 800-279-6799, 602-265-2651, FAX: 602-265-2650, 800-279-4663. PRICE: $49.50. ISBN: 157356110X.

Summary: This book provides information on schools and programs in the United States and Canada that offer professional training in alternative and complementary modalities, including acupressure, acupuncture, Alexander technique, **aromatherapy,** Ayurvedic medicine, biofeedback, chiropractic, Feldenkrais, herbal medicine, homeopathy, hypnotherapy, massage therapy and bodywork, midwifery, naturopathic medicine, Oriental medicine, polarity therapy, reflexology, reiki, Shiatsu, and yoga. The book contains a list of abbreviations, a glossary, a subject index, and nine essays on selected alternative medicine health fields describing each modality and the training and education required to practice in that field. The alphabetical listing of schools by state provides contact information, including the school's name, address, telephone number, fax number, e-mail address, and Web page address, if available. The school listing is followed by a list of organizations and accrediting bodies and resources for further reading. This book also provides an index of schools by name and by specialization, and a general index.

---

the bottom of the search page where "You may refine your search by." For publication date, select "All Years." Select your preferred language and the format option "Directory." Type "aromatherapy" (or synonyms) into the "For these words:" box. You should check back periodically with this database as it is updated every three months.

CHAPTER 6. MULTIMEDIA ON AROMATHERAPY

Overview

In this chapter, we show you how to keep current on multimedia sources of information on aromatherapy. We start with sources that have been summarized by federal agencies, and then show you how to find bibliographic information catalogued by the National Library of Medicine.

Bibliography: Multimedia on Aromatherapy

The National Library of Medicine is a rich source of information on healthcare-related multimedia productions including slides, computer software, and databases. To access the multimedia database, go to the following Web site: **http://locatorplus.gov/**. Select "Search LOCATORplus." Once in the search area, simply type in aromatherapy (or synonyms). Then, in the option box provided below the search box, select "Audiovisuals and Computer Files." From there, you can choose to sort results by publication date, author, or relevance. The following multimedia has been indexed on aromatherapy (for more information, follow the hyperlink indicated):

- **Aromatherapy [videorecording]: the therapeutic effects of essential oils** Source: VisionQuest Video; Year: 1995; Format: Videorecording; [Australia]: MPI Productions; Buffalo, NY: Kinetic [distributor], c1995

- **Genusys [electronic resource]: database of herbal remedies, aromatherapy, essential oils, vitamins, amino acids, and more!** Year: 1996; Format: Electronic resource; Solebury, PA: Genusys Laboratories, c1996

- **Holistic aromatherapy training [videorecording]** Source: produced by Talking Pictures, Ltd; Year: 2002; Format: Videorecording; Derry, N.H.: Chip Taylor Communications, 2002

CHAPTER 7. PERIODICALS AND NEWS ON AROMATHERAPY

Overview

In this chapter, we suggest a number of news sources and present various periodicals that cover aromatherapy.

News Services and Press Releases

One of the simplest ways of tracking press releases on aromatherapy is to search the news wires. In the following sample of sources, we will briefly describe how to access each service. These services only post recent news intended for public viewing.

PR Newswire

To access the PR Newswire archive, simply go to **http://www.prnewswire.com/**. Select your country. Type "aromatherapy" (or synonyms) into the search box. You will automatically receive information on relevant news releases posted within the last 30 days. The search results are shown by order of relevance.

Reuters Health

The Reuters' Medical News and Health eLine databases can be very useful in exploring news archives relating to aromatherapy. While some of the listed articles are free to view, others are available for purchase for a nominal fee. To access this archive, go to **http://www.reutershealth.com/en/index.html** and search by "aromatherapy" (or synonyms). The following was recently listed in this archive for aromatherapy:

- **Light, aromatherapy help dementia patients**
  Source: Reuters Health eLine
  Date: August 19, 2003

- **Aromatherapy may be useful for dementia patients**
  Source: Reuters Health eLine
  Date: December 06, 2002

- **Aromatherapy may be beneficial for dementia patients**
  Source: Reuters Medical News
  Date: December 06, 2002

- **Aromatherapy safe and effective treatment of agitation among dementia patients**
  Source: Reuters Medical News
  Date: August 23, 2002

- **Aromatherapy soothes agitation in the demented**
  Source: Reuters Health eLine
  Date: August 07, 2002

- **Study results do not back aromatherapy claims**
  Source: Reuters Health eLine
  Date: July 03, 2000

- **Aromatherapy helps temporary hair loss**
  Source: Reuters Health eLine
  Date: December 17, 1998

The NIH

Within MEDLINEplus, the NIH has made an agreement with the New York Times Syndicate, the AP News Service, and Reuters to deliver news that can be browsed by the public. Search news releases at **http://www.nlm.nih.gov/medlineplus/alphanews_a.html**. MEDLINEplus allows you to browse across an alphabetical index. Or you can search by date at the following Web page: **http://www.nlm.nih.gov/medlineplus/newsbydate.html**. Often, news items are indexed by MEDLINEplus within its search engine.

Business Wire

Business Wire is similar to PR Newswire. To access this archive, simply go to **http://www.businesswire.com/**. You can scan the news by industry category or company name.

Market Wire

Market Wire is more focused on technology than the other wires. To browse the latest press releases by topic, such as alternative medicine, biotechnology, fitness, healthcare, legal, nutrition, and pharmaceuticals, access Market Wire's Medical/Health channel at **http://www.marketwire.com/mw/release_index?channel=MedicalHealth**. Or simply go to Market Wire's home page at **http://www.marketwire.com/mw/home**, type "aromatherapy" (or synonyms) into the search box, and click on "Search News." As this service is technology oriented, you may wish to use it when searching for press releases covering diagnostic procedures or tests.

Search Engines

Medical news is also available in the news sections of commercial Internet search engines. See the health news page at Yahoo (**http://dir.yahoo.com/Health/News_and_Media/**), or you can use this Web site's general news search page at **http://news.yahoo.com/**. Type in "aromatherapy" (or synonyms). If you know the name of a company that is relevant to aromatherapy, you can go to any stock trading Web site (such as **http://www.etrade.com/**) and search for the company name there. News items across various news sources are reported on indicated hyperlinks. Google offers a similar service at **http://news.google.com/**.

BBC

Covering news from a more European perspective, the British Broadcasting Corporation (BBC) allows the public free access to their news archive located at **http://www.bbc.co.uk/**. Search by "aromatherapy" (or synonyms).

Academic Periodicals covering Aromatherapy

Numerous periodicals are currently indexed within the National Library of Medicine's PubMed database that are known to publish articles relating to aromatherapy. In addition to these sources, you can search for articles covering aromatherapy that have been published by any of the periodicals listed in previous chapters. To find the latest studies published, go to **http://www.ncbi.nlm.nih.gov/pubmed**, type the name of the periodical into the search box, and click "Go."

If you want complete details about the historical contents of a journal, you can also visit the following Web site: **http://www.ncbi.nlm.nih.gov/entrez/jrbrowser.cgi**. Here, type in the name of the journal or its abbreviation, and you will receive an index of published articles. At **http://locatorplus.gov/**, you can retrieve more indexing information on medical periodicals (e.g. the name of the publisher). Select the button "Search LOCATORplus." Then type in the name of the journal and select the advanced search option "Journal Title Search."

APPENDICES

APPENDIX A. PHYSICIAN RESOURCES

Overview

In this chapter, we focus on databases and Internet-based guidelines and information resources created or written for a professional audience.

NIH Guidelines

Commonly referred to as "clinical" or "professional" guidelines, the National Institutes of Health publish physician guidelines for the most common diseases. Publications are available at the following by relevant Institute[9]:

- Office of the Director (OD); guidelines consolidated across agencies available at **http://www.nih.gov/health/consumer/conkey.htm**

- National Institute of General Medical Sciences (NIGMS); fact sheets available at **http://www.nigms.nih.gov/news/facts/**

- National Library of Medicine (NLM); extensive encyclopedia (A.D.A.M., Inc.) with guidelines: **http://www.nlm.nih.gov/medlineplus/healthtopics.html**

- National Cancer Institute (NCI); guidelines available at **http://www.cancer.gov/cancerinfo/list.aspx?viewid=5f35036e-5497-4d86-8c2c-714a9f7c8d25**

- National Eye Institute (NEI); guidelines available at **http://www.nei.nih.gov/order/index.htm**

- National Heart, Lung, and Blood Institute (NHLBI); guidelines available at **http://www.nhlbi.nih.gov/guidelines/index.htm**

- National Human Genome Research Institute (NHGRI); research available at **http://www.genome.gov/page.cfm?pageID=10000375**

- National Institute on Aging (NIA); guidelines available at **http://www.nia.nih.gov/health/**

---

[9] These publications are typically written by one or more of the various NIH Institutes.

- National Institute on Alcohol Abuse and Alcoholism (NIAAA); guidelines available at **http://www.niaaa.nih.gov/publications/publications.htm**

- National Institute of Allergy and Infectious Diseases (NIAID); guidelines available at **http://www.niaid.nih.gov/publications/**

- National Institute of Arthritis and Musculoskeletal and Skin Diseases (NIAMS); fact sheets and guidelines available at **http://www.niams.nih.gov/hi/index.htm**

- National Institute of Child Health and Human Development (NICHD); guidelines available at **http://www.nichd.nih.gov/publications/pubskey.cfm**

- National Institute on Deafness and Other Communication Disorders (NIDCD); fact sheets and guidelines at **http://www.nidcd.nih.gov/health/**

- National Institute of Dental and Craniofacial Research (NIDCR); guidelines available at **http://www.nidr.nih.gov/health/**

- National Institute of Diabetes and Digestive and Kidney Diseases (NIDDK); guidelines available at **http://www.niddk.nih.gov/health/health.htm**

- National Institute on Drug Abuse (NIDA); guidelines available at **http://www.nida.nih.gov/DrugAbuse.html**

- National Institute of Environmental Health Sciences (NIEHS); environmental health information available at **http://www.niehs.nih.gov/external/facts.htm**

- National Institute of Mental Health (NIMH); guidelines available at **http://www.nimh.nih.gov/practitioners/index.cfm**

- National Institute of Neurological Disorders and Stroke (NINDS); neurological disorder information pages available at **http://www.ninds.nih.gov/health_and_medical/disorder_index.htm**

- National Institute of Nursing Research (NINR); publications on selected illnesses at **http://www.nih.gov/ninr/news-info/publications.html**

- National Institute of Biomedical Imaging and Bioengineering; general information at **http://grants.nih.gov/grants/becon/becon_info.htm**

- Center for Information Technology (CIT); referrals to other agencies based on keyword searches available at **http://kb.nih.gov/www_query_main.asp**

- National Center for Complementary and Alternative Medicine (NCCAM); health information available at **http://nccam.nih.gov/health/**

- National Center for Research Resources (NCRR); various information directories available at **http://www.ncrr.nih.gov/publications.asp**

- Office of Rare Diseases; various fact sheets available at **http://rarediseases.info.nih.gov/html/resources/rep_pubs.html**

- Centers for Disease Control and Prevention; various fact sheets on infectious diseases available at **http://www.cdc.gov/publications.htm**

NIH Databases

In addition to the various Institutes of Health that publish professional guidelines, the NIH has designed a number of databases for professionals.[10] Physician-oriented resources provide a wide variety of information related to the biomedical and health sciences, both past and present. The format of these resources varies. Searchable databases, bibliographic citations, full-text articles (when available), archival collections, and images are all available. The following are referenced by the National Library of Medicine:[11]

- **Bioethics:** Access to published literature on the ethical, legal, and public policy issues surrounding healthcare and biomedical research. This information is provided in conjunction with the Kennedy Institute of Ethics located at Georgetown University, Washington, D.C.: **http://www.nlm.nih.gov/databases/databases_bioethics.html**

- **HIV/AIDS Resources:** Describes various links and databases dedicated to HIV/AIDS research: **http://www.nlm.nih.gov/pubs/factsheets/aidsinfs.html**

- **NLM Online Exhibitions:** Describes "Exhibitions in the History of Medicine": **http://www.nlm.nih.gov/exhibition/exhibition.html**. Additional resources for historical scholarship in medicine: **http://www.nlm.nih.gov/hmd/hmd.html**

- **Biotechnology Information:** Access to public databases. The National Center for Biotechnology Information conducts research in computational biology, develops software tools for analyzing genome data, and disseminates biomedical information for the better understanding of molecular processes affecting human health and disease: **http://www.ncbi.nlm.nih.gov/**

- **Population Information:** The National Library of Medicine provides access to worldwide coverage of population, family planning, and related health issues, including family planning technology and programs, fertility, and population law and policy: **http://www.nlm.nih.gov/databases/databases_population.html**

- **Cancer Information:** Access to cancer-oriented databases: **http://www.nlm.nih.gov/databases/databases_cancer.html**

- **Profiles in Science:** Offering the archival collections of prominent twentieth-century biomedical scientists to the public through modern digital technology: **http://www.profiles.nlm.nih.gov/**

- **Chemical Information:** Provides links to various chemical databases and references: **http://sis.nlm.nih.gov/Chem/ChemMain.html**

- **Clinical Alerts:** Reports the release of findings from the NIH-funded clinical trials where such release could significantly affect morbidity and mortality: **http://www.nlm.nih.gov/databases/alerts/clinical_alerts.html**

- **Space Life Sciences:** Provides links and information to space-based research (including NASA): **http://www.nlm.nih.gov/databases/databases_space.html**

- **MEDLINE:** Bibliographic database covering the fields of medicine, nursing, dentistry, veterinary medicine, the healthcare system, and the pre-clinical sciences: **http://www.nlm.nih.gov/databases/databases_medline.html**

---

[10] Remember, for the general public, the National Library of Medicine recommends the databases referenced in MEDLINE*plus* (**http://medlineplus.gov/** or **http://www.nlm.nih.gov/medlineplus/databases.html**).

[11] See **http://www.nlm.nih.gov/databases/databases.html**.

- **Toxicology and Environmental Health Information (TOXNET):** Databases covering toxicology and environmental health: **http://sis.nlm.nih.gov/Tox/ToxMain.html**

- **Visible Human Interface:** Anatomically detailed, three-dimensional representations of normal male and female human bodies: **http://www.nlm.nih.gov/research/visible/visible_human.html**

The NLM Gateway[12]

The NLM (National Library of Medicine) Gateway is a Web-based system that lets users search simultaneously in multiple retrieval systems at the U.S. National Library of Medicine (NLM). It allows users of NLM services to initiate searches from one Web interface, providing one-stop searching for many of NLM's information resources or databases.[13] To use the NLM Gateway, simply go to the search site at **http://gateway.nlm.nih.gov/gw/Cmd**. Type "aromatherapy" (or synonyms) into the search box and click "Search." The results will be presented in a tabular form, indicating the number of references in each database category.

Results Summary

Category	Items Found
Journal Articles	290
Books / Periodicals / Audio Visual	60
Consumer Health	1
Meeting Abstracts	4
Other Collections	0
Total	355

HSTAT[14]

HSTAT is a free, Web-based resource that provides access to full-text documents used in healthcare decision-making.[15] These documents include clinical practice guidelines, quick-reference guides for clinicians, consumer health brochures, evidence reports and technology assessments from the Agency for Healthcare Research and Quality (AHRQ), as well as AHRQ's Put Prevention Into Practice.[16] Simply search by "aromatherapy" (or synonyms) at the following Web site: **http://text.nlm.nih.gov**.

---

[12] Adapted from NLM: **http://gateway.nlm.nih.gov/gw/Cmd?Overview.x**

[13] The NLM Gateway is currently being developed by the Lister Hill National Center for Biomedical Communications (LHNCBC) at the National Library of Medicine (NLM) of the National Institutes of Health (NIH).

[14] Adapted from HSTAT: **http://www.nlm.nih.gov/pubs/factsheets/hstat.html**.

[15] The HSTAT URL is **http://hstat.nlm.nih.gov/**.

[16] Other important documents in HSTAT include: the National Institutes of Health (NIH) Consensus Conference Reports and Technology Assessment Reports; the HIV/AIDS Treatment Information Service (ATIS) resource documents; the Substance Abuse and Mental Health Services Administration's Center for Substance Abuse Treatment (SAMHSA/CSAT) Treatment Improvement Protocols (TIP) and Center for Substance Abuse Prevention (SAMHSA/CSAP) Prevention Enhancement Protocols System (PEPS); the Public Health Service (PHS) Preventive Services Task Force's *Guide to Clinical Preventive Services*; the independent, nonfederal Task Force on Community Services' *Guide to Community Preventive Services*; and the Health Technology Advisory Committee (HTAC) of the Minnesota Health Care Commission (MHCC) health technology evaluations.

Coffee Break: Tutorials for Biologists [17]

Coffee Break is a general healthcare site that takes a scientific view of the news and covers recent breakthroughs in biology that may one day assist physicians in developing treatments. Here you will find a collection of short reports on recent biological discoveries. Each report incorporates interactive tutorials that demonstrate how bioinformatics tools are used as a part of the research process. Currently, all Coffee Breaks are written by NCBI staff. [18] Each report is about 400 words and is usually based on a discovery reported in one or more articles from recently published, peer-reviewed literature. [19] This site has new articles every few weeks, so it can be considered an online magazine of sorts. It is intended for general background information. You can access the Coffee Break Web site at the following hyperlink: **http://www.ncbi.nlm.nih.gov/Coffeebreak/**.

Other Commercial Databases

In addition to resources maintained by official agencies, other databases exist that are commercial ventures addressing medical professionals. Here are some examples that may interest you:

- **CliniWeb International:** Index and table of contents to selected clinical information on the Internet; see **http://www.ohsu.edu/cliniweb/**.

- **Medical World Search:** Searches full text from thousands of selected medical sites on the Internet; see **http://www.mwsearch.com/**.

---

[17] Adapted from **http://www.ncbi.nlm.nih.gov/Coffeebreak/Archive/FAQ.html**.

[18] The figure that accompanies each article is frequently supplied by an expert external to NCBI, in which case the source of the figure is cited. The result is an interactive tutorial that tells a biological story.

[19] After a brief introduction that sets the work described into a broader context, the report focuses on how a molecular understanding can provide explanations of observed biology and lead to therapies for diseases. Each vignette is accompanied by a figure and hypertext links that lead to a series of pages that interactively show how NCBI tools and resources are used in the research process.

APPENDIX B. PATIENT RESOURCES

Overview

Official agencies, as well as federally funded institutions supported by national grants, frequently publish a variety of guidelines written with the patient in mind. These are typically called "Fact Sheets" or "Guidelines." They can take the form of a brochure, information kit, pamphlet, or flyer. Often they are only a few pages in length. Since new guidelines on aromatherapy can appear at any moment and be published by a number of sources, the best approach to finding guidelines is to systematically scan the Internet-based services that post them.

Patient Guideline Sources

The remainder of this chapter directs you to sources which either publish or can help you find additional guidelines on topics related to aromatherapy. Due to space limitations, these sources are listed in a concise manner. Do not hesitate to consult the following sources by either using the Internet hyperlink provided, or, in cases where the contact information is provided, contacting the publisher or author directly.

The National Institutes of Health

The NIH gateway to patients is located at **http://health.nih.gov/**. From this site, you can search across various sources and institutes, a number of which are summarized below.

Topic Pages: MEDLINEplus

The National Library of Medicine has created a vast and patient-oriented healthcare information portal called MEDLINEplus. Within this Internet-based system are "health topic pages" which list links to available materials relevant to aromatherapy. To access this system, log on to **http://www.nlm.nih.gov/medlineplus/healthtopics.html**. From there you can either search using the alphabetical index or browse by broad topic areas. Recently, MEDLINEplus listed the following when searched for "aromatherapy":

- Other guides

    About Your Medicines
    http://www.nlm.nih.gov/medlineplus/aboutyourmedicines.html

    Arthritis
    http://www.nlm.nih.gov/medlineplus/arthritis.html

    Cancer Alternative Therapy
    http://www.nlm.nih.gov/medlineplus/canceralternativetherapy.html

    Environmental Health
    http://www.nlm.nih.gov/medlineplus/environmentalhealth.html

    Hepatitis C
    http://www.nlm.nih.gov/medlineplus/hepatitisc.html

    Herbal Medicine
    http://www.nlm.nih.gov/medlineplus/herbalmedicine.html

    Household Poisons
    http://www.nlm.nih.gov/medlineplus/householdpoisons.html

You may also choose to use the search utility provided by MEDLINEplus at the following Web address: **http://www.nlm.nih.gov/medlineplus/**. Simply type a keyword into the search box and click "Search." This utility is similar to the NIH search utility, with the exception that it only includes materials that are linked within the MEDLINEplus system (mostly patient-oriented information). It also has the disadvantage of generating unstructured results. We recommend, therefore, that you use this method only if you have a very targeted search.

The Combined Health Information Database (CHID)

CHID Online is a reference tool that maintains a database directory of thousands of journal articles and patient education guidelines on aromatherapy. CHID offers summaries that describe the guidelines available, including contact information and pricing. CHID's general Web site is **http://chid.nih.gov/**. To search this database, go to **http://chid.nih.gov/detail/detail.html**. In particular, you can use the advanced search options to look up pamphlets, reports, brochures, and information kits. The following was recently posted in this archive:

- **A Practical Guide to Complementary Therapies for People Living With HIV**

    Contact: Community AIDS Treatment Information Exchange, PO Box 1104, Toronto, (416) 203-7122, http://www.catie.ca.

    Summary: This brochure discusses the use of complementary therapies for persons with the human immunodeficiency virus (HIV). It discusses research and complementary therapies; the regulation of practitioners; several therapeutic systems including Ayurvedic medicine, homeopathy, North American Aboriginal healing traditions, naturopathy, and traditional Chinese medicine (TCM); several wellness systems including **aromatherapy,** color therapy, and juicing; unconventional therapies using melatonin and oxygen; and how to find a practicioner and avoid health fraud.

- **[Introduction to Complementary Therapies]**

  Contact: Canadian Public Health Association, Canadian HIV/AIDS Clearinghouse, 400-1565 Carling Ave Ste 400, Ottawa, (613) 725-3434, http://www.cpha.ca.

  Summary: This pamphlet discusses complementary therapies that may help the patient with human immunodeficiency virus (HIV)/acquired immunodeficiency disease (AIDS). The pamphlet compares western medicine and complementary therapies and describes the following therapies: ayurveda, acupuncture and acupressure, **aromatherapy,** chiropractic therapy, massage, meditation, naturopathy, reflexology, reiki, shiatsu massage, sidha medicine, tai chi, and yoga. The pamphlet advises the patient to consult the physician about therapies he/she plans to take and to inform the complementary therapist about prescribed drugs being taken.

- **Coping with Hepatitis C: Alternative or Complementary Approaches**

  Source: San Francisco, CA: National Hepatitis C Program, Department of Veterans Affairs Medical Center. 2002. 3 p.

  Contact: Available from National Hepatitis C Program. Department of Veterans Affairs Medical Center, 4150 Clement Street, San Francisco, CA 94121. (415) 750-2105. PRICE: Free.

  Summary: This patient education brochure from the Centers of Excellence in Hepatitis C Research and Education at the Veterans Administration provides information about complementary and alternative medicine (CAM) approaches for people who have hepatitis C. It lists three guidelines to follow if alternative treatments will be used, and gives important warnings about herbal remedies, supplements, vitamins, and other natural treatments. It also discusses several types of CAM treatments for hepatitis C, including **aromatherapy,** massage therapy, meditation and visualization, and yoga.

Healthfinder™

Healthfinder™ is sponsored by the U.S. Department of Health and Human Services and offers links to hundreds of other sites that contain healthcare information. This Web site is located at **http://www.healthfinder.gov**. Again, keyword searches can be used to find guidelines. The following was recently found in this database:

- **Aromatherapy - Frequently Asked Questions**

  Summary: Provides answers to questions about aromatherapy.

  Source: NOAH: New York Online Access to Health

  http://www.healthfinder.gov/scripts/recordpass.asp?RecordType=0&RecordID=7355

The NIH Search Utility

The NIH search utility allows you to search for documents on over 100 selected Web sites that comprise the NIH-WEB-SPACE. Each of these servers is "crawled" and indexed on an ongoing basis. Your search will produce a list of various documents, all of which will relate in some way to aromatherapy. The drawbacks of this approach are that the information is not organized by theme and that the references are often a mix of information for professionals and patients. Nevertheless, a large number of the listed Web sites provide useful background information. We can only recommend this route, therefore, for relatively rare or specific disorders, or when using highly targeted searches. To use the NIH search utility, visit the following Web page: **http://search.nih.gov/index.html**

Additional Web Sources

A number of Web sites are available to the public that often link to government sites. These can also point you in the direction of essential information. The following is a representative sample:

- AOL: **http://search.aol.com/cat.adp?id=168&layer=&from=subcats**

- Family Village: **http://www.familyvillage.wisc.edu/specific.htm**

- Google: **http://directory.google.com/Top/Health/Conditions_and_Diseases/**

- Med Help International: **http://www.medhelp.org/HealthTopics/A.html**

- Open Directory Project: **http://dmoz.org/Health/Conditions_and_Diseases/**

- Yahoo.com: **http://dir.yahoo.com/Health/Diseases_and_Conditions/**

- WebMD®Health: **http://my.webmd.com/health_topics**

Finding Associations

There are several Internet directories that provide lists of medical associations with information on or resources relating to aromatherapy. By consulting all of associations listed in this chapter, you will have nearly exhausted all sources for patient associations concerned with aromatherapy.

The National Health Information Center (NHIC)

The National Health Information Center (NHIC) offers a free referral service to help people find organizations that provide information about aromatherapy. For more information, see the NHIC's Web site at **http://www.health.gov/NHIC/** or contact an information specialist by calling 1-800-336-4797.

Directory of Health Organizations

The Directory of Health Organizations, provided by the National Library of Medicine Specialized Information Services, is a comprehensive source of information on associations. The Directory of Health Organizations database can be accessed via the Internet at **http://www.sis.nlm.nih.gov/Dir/DirMain.html**. It is composed of two parts: DIRLINE and Health Hotlines.

The DIRLINE database comprises some 10,000 records of organizations, research centers, and government institutes and associations that primarily focus on health and biomedicine. To access DIRLINE directly, go to the following Web site: **http://dirline.nlm.nih.gov/**. Simply type in "aromatherapy" (or a synonym), and you will receive information on all relevant organizations listed in the database.

Health Hotlines directs you to toll-free numbers to over 300 organizations. You can access this database directly at **http://www.sis.nlm.nih.gov/hotlines/**. On this page, you are given the option to search by keyword or by browsing the subject list. When you have received your search results, click on the name of the organization for its description and contact information.

The Combined Health Information Database

Another comprehensive source of information on healthcare associations is the Combined Health Information Database. Using the "Detailed Search" option, you will need to limit your search to "Organizations" and "aromatherapy". Type the following hyperlink into your Web browser: **http://chid.nih.gov/detail/detail.html**. To find associations, use the drop boxes at the bottom of the search page where "You may refine your search by." For publication date, select "All Years." Then, select your preferred language and the format option "Organization Resource Sheet." Type "aromatherapy" (or synonyms) into the "For these words:" box. You should check back periodically with this database since it is updated every three months.

The National Organization for Rare Disorders, Inc.

The National Organization for Rare Disorders, Inc. has prepared a Web site that provides, at no charge, lists of associations organized by health topic. You can access this database at the following Web site: **http://www.rarediseases.org/search/orgsearch.html**. Type "aromatherapy" (or a synonym) into the search box, and click "Submit Query."

APPENDIX C. FINDING MEDICAL LIBRARIES

Overview

In this Appendix, we show you how to quickly find a medical library in your area.

Preparation

Your local public library and medical libraries have interlibrary loan programs with the National Library of Medicine (NLM), one of the largest medical collections in the world. According to the NLM, most of the literature in the general and historical collections of the National Library of Medicine is available on interlibrary loan to any library. If you would like to access NLM medical literature, then visit a library in your area that can request the publications for you.[20]

Finding a Local Medical Library

The quickest method to locate medical libraries is to use the Internet-based directory published by the National Network of Libraries of Medicine (NN/LM). This network includes 4626 members and affiliates that provide many services to librarians, health professionals, and the public. To find a library in your area, simply visit **http://nnlm.gov/members/adv.html** or call 1-800-338-7657.

Medical Libraries in the U.S. and Canada

In addition to the NN/LM, the National Library of Medicine (NLM) lists a number of libraries with reference facilities that are open to the public. The following is the NLM's list and includes hyperlinks to each library's Web site. These Web pages can provide information on hours of operation and other restrictions. The list below is a small sample of

---

[20] Adapted from the NLM: **http://www.nlm.nih.gov/psd/cas/inte library.html**.

libraries recommended by the National Library of Medicine (sorted alphabetically by name of the U.S. state or Canadian province where the library is located)[21]:

- **Alabama:** Health InfoNet of Jefferson County (Jefferson County Library Cooperative, Lister Hill Library of the Health Sciences), **http://www.uab.edu/infonet/**

- **Alabama:** Richard M. Scrushy Library (American Sports Medicine Institute)

- **Arizona:** Samaritan Regional Medical Center: The Learning Center (Samaritan Health System, Phoenix, Arizona), **http://www.samaritan.edu/library/bannerlibs.htm**

- **California:** Kris Kelly Health Information Center (St. Joseph Health System, Humboldt), **http://www.humboldt1.com/~kkhic/index.html**

- **California:** Community Health Library of Los Gatos, **http://www.healthlib.org/orgresources.html**

- **California:** Consumer Health Program and Services (CHIPS) (County of Los Angeles Public Library, Los Angeles County Harbor-UCLA Medical Center Library) - Carson, CA, **http://www.colapublib.org/services/chips.html**

- **California:** Gateway Health Library (Sutter Gould Medical Foundation)

- **California:** Health Library (Stanford University Medical Center), **http://www-med.stanford.edu/healthlibrary/**

- **California:** Patient Education Resource Center - Health Information and Resources (University of California, San Francisco), **http://sfghdean.ucsf.edu/barnett/PERC/default.asp**

- **California:** Redwood Health Library (Petaluma Health Care District), **http://www.phcd.org/rdwdlib.html**

- **California:** Los Gatos PlaneTree Health Library, **http://planetreesanjose.org/**

- **California:** Sutter Resource Library (Sutter Hospitals Foundation, Sacramento), **http://suttermedicalcenter.org/library/**

- **California:** Health Sciences Libraries (University of California, Davis), **http://www.lib.ucdavis.edu/healthsci/**

- **California:** ValleyCare Health Library & Ryan Comer Cancer Resource Center (ValleyCare Health System, Pleasanton), **http://gaelnet.stmarys-ca.edu/other.libs/gbal/east/vchl.html**

- **California:** Washington Community Health Resource Library (Fremont), **http://www.healthlibrary.org/**

- **Colorado:** William V. Gervasini Memorial Library (Exempla Healthcare), **http://www.saintjosephdenver.org/yourhealth/libraries/**

- **Connecticut:** Hartford Hospital Health Science Libraries (Hartford Hospital), **http://www.harthosp.org/library/**

- **Connecticut:** Healthnet: Connecticut Consumer Health Information Center (University of Connecticut Health Center, Lyman Maynard Stowe Library), **http://library.uchc.edu/departm/hnet/**

---

[21] Abstracted from **http://www.nlm.nih.gov/medlineplus/libraries.html**.

- **Connecticut:** Waterbury Hospital Health Center Library (Waterbury Hospital, Waterbury), **http://www.waterburyhospital.com/library/consumer.shtml**

- **Delaware:** Consumer Health Library (Christiana Care Health System, Eugene du Pont Preventive Medicine & Rehabilitation Institute, Wilmington), **http://www.christianacare.org/health_guide/health_guide_pmri_health_info.cfm**

- **Delaware:** Lewis B. Flinn Library (Delaware Academy of Medicine, Wilmington), **http://www.delamed.org/chls.html**

- **Georgia:** Family Resource Library (Medical College of Georgia, Augusta), **http://cmc.mcg.edu/kids_families/fam_resources/fam_res_lib/frl.htm**

- **Georgia:** Health Resource Center (Medical Center of Central Georgia, Macon), **http://www.mccg.org/hrc/hrchome.asp**

- **Hawaii:** Hawaii Medical Library: Consumer Health Information Service (Hawaii Medical Library, Honolulu), **http://hml.org/CHIS/**

- **Idaho:** DeArmond Consumer Health Library (Kootenai Medical Center, Coeur d'Alene), **http://www.nicon.org/DeArmond/index.htm**

- **Illinois:** Health Learning Center of Northwestern Memorial Hospital (Chicago), **http://www.nmh.org/health_info/hlc.html**

- **Illinois:** Medical Library (OSF Saint Francis Medical Center, Peoria), **http://www.osfsaintfrancis.org/general/library/**

- **Kentucky:** Medical Library - Services for Patients, Families, Students & the Public (Central Baptist Hospital, Lexington), **http://www.centralbap.com/education/community/library.cfm**

- **Kentucky:** University of Kentucky - Health Information Library (Chandler Medical Center, Lexington), **http://www.mc.uky.edu/PatientEd/**

- **Louisiana:** Alton Ochsner Medical Foundation Library (Alton Ochsner Medical Foundation, New Orleans), **http://www.ochsner.org/library/**

- **Louisiana:** Louisiana State University Health Sciences Center Medical Library-Shreveport, **http://lib-sh.lsuhsc.edu/**

- **Maine:** Franklin Memorial Hospital Medical Library (Franklin Memorial Hospital, Farmington), **http://www.fchn.org/fmh/lib.htm**

- **Maine:** Gerrish-True Health Sciences Library (Central Maine Medical Center, Lewiston), **http://www.cmmc.org/library/library.html**

- **Maine:** Hadley Parrot Health Science Library (Eastern Maine Healthcare, Bangor), **http://www.emh.org/hll/hpl/guide.htm**

- **Maine:** Maine Medical Center Library (Maine Medical Center, Portland), **http://www.mmc.org/library/**

- **Maine:** Parkview Hospital (Brunswick), **http://www.parkviewhospital.org/**

- **Maine:** Southern Maine Medical Center Health Sciences Library (Southern Maine Medical Center, Biddeford), **http://www.smmc.org/services/service.php3?choice=10**

- **Maine:** Stephens Memorial Hospital's Health Information Library (Western Maine Health, Norway), **http://www.wmhcc.org/Library/**

- **Manitoba, Canada:** Consumer & Patient Health Information Service (University of Manitoba Libraries), **http://www.umanitoba.ca/libraries/units/health/reference/chis.html**

- **Manitoba, Canada:** J.W. Crane Memorial Library (Deer Lodge Centre, Winnipeg), **http://www.deerlodge.mb.ca/crane_library/about.asp**

- **Maryland:** Health Information Center at the Wheaton Regional Library (Montgomery County, Dept. of Public Libraries, Wheaton Regional Library), **http://www.mont.lib.md.us/healthinfo/hic.asp**

- **Massachusetts:** Baystate Medical Center Library (Baystate Health System), **http://www.baystatehealth.com/1024/**

- **Massachusetts:** Boston University Medical Center Alumni Medical Library (Boston University Medical Center), **http://med-libwww.bu.edu/library/lib.html**

- **Massachusetts:** Lowell General Hospital Health Sciences Library (Lowell General Hospital, Lowell), **http://www.lowellgeneral.org/library/HomePageLinks/WWW.htm**

- **Massachusetts:** Paul E. Woodard Health Sciences Library (New England Baptist Hospital, Boston), **http://www.nebh.org/health_lib.asp**

- **Massachusetts:** St. Luke's Hospital Health Sciences Library (St. Luke's Hospital, Southcoast Health System, New Bedford), **http://www.southcoast.org/library/**

- **Massachusetts:** Treadwell Library Consumer Health Reference Center (Massachusetts General Hospital), **http://www.mgh.harvard.edu/library/chrcindex.html**

- **Massachusetts:** UMass HealthNet (University of Massachusetts Medical School, Worchester), **http://healthnet.umassmed.edu/**

- **Michigan:** Botsford General Hospital Library - Consumer Health (Botsford General Hospital, Library & Internet Services), **http://www.botsfordlibrary.org/consumer.htm**

- **Michigan:** Helen DeRoy Medical Library (Providence Hospital and Medical Centers), **http://www.providence-hospital.org/library/**

- **Michigan:** Marquette General Hospital - Consumer Health Library (Marquette General Hospital, Health Information Center), **http://www.mgh.org/center.html**

- **Michigan:** Patient Education Resouce Center - University of Michigan Cancer Center (University of Michigan Comprehensive Cancer Center, Ann Arbor), **http://www.cancer.med.umich.edu/learn/leares.htm**

- **Michigan:** Sladen Library & Center for Health Information Resources - Consumer Health Information (Detroit), **http://www.henryford.com/body.cfm?id=39330**

- **Montana:** Center for Health Information (St. Patrick Hospital and Health Sciences Center, Missoula)

- **National:** Consumer Health Library Directory (Medical Library Association, Consumer and Patient Health Information Section), **http://caphis.mlanet.org/directory/index.html**

- **National:** National Network of Libraries of Medicine (National Library of Medicine) - provides library services for health professionals in the United States who do not have access to a medical library, **http://nnlm.gov/**

- **National:** NN/LM List of Libraries Serving the Public (National Network of Libraries of Medicine), **http://nnlm.gov/members/**

- **Nevada:** Health Science Library, West Charleston Library (Las Vegas-Clark County Library District, Las Vegas), **http://www.lvccld.org/special_collections/medical/index.htm**

- **New Hampshire:** Dartmouth Biomedical Libraries (Dartmouth College Library, Hanover), **http://www.dartmouth.edu/~biomed/resources.htmld/conshealth.htmld/**

- **New Jersey:** Consumer Health Library (Rahway Hospital, Rahway), **http://www.rahwayhospital.com/library.htm**

- **New Jersey:** Dr. Walter Phillips Health Sciences Library (Englewood Hospital and Medical Center, Englewood), **http://www.englewoodhospital.com/links/index.htm**

- **New Jersey:** Meland Foundation (Englewood Hospital and Medical Center, Englewood), **http://www.geocities.com/ResearchTriangle/9360/**

- **New York:** Choices in Health Information (New York Public Library) - NLM Consumer Pilot Project participant, **http://www.nypl.org/branch/health/links.html**

- **New York:** Health Information Center (Upstate Medical University, State University of New York, Syracuse), **http://www.upstate.edu/library/hic/**

- **New York:** Health Sciences Library (Long Island Jewish Medical Center, New Hyde Park), **http://www.lij.edu/library/library.html**

- **New York:** ViaHealth Medical Library (Rochester General Hospital), **http://www.nyam.org/library/**

- **Ohio:** Consumer Health Library (Akron General Medical Center, Medical & Consumer Health Library), **http://www.akrongeneral.org/hwlibrary.htm**

- **Oklahoma:** The Health Information Center at Saint Francis Hospital (Saint Francis Health System, Tulsa), **http://www.sfh-tulsa.com/services/healthinfo.asp**

- **Oregon:** Planetree Health Resource Center (Mid-Columbia Medical Center, The Dalles), **http://www.mcmc.net/phrc/**

- **Pennsylvania:** Community Health Information Library (Milton S. Hershey Medical Center, Hershey), **http://www.hmc.psu.edu/commhealth/**

- **Pennsylvania:** Community Health Resource Library (Geisinger Medical Center, Danville), **http://www.geisinger.edu/education/commlib.shtml**

- **Pennsylvania:** HealthInfo Library (Moses Taylor Hospital, Scranton), **http://www.mth.org/healthwellness.html**

- **Pennsylvania:** Hopwood Library (University of Pittsburgh, Health Sciences Library System, Pittsburgh), **http://www.hsls.pitt.edu/guides/chi/hopwood/index_html**

- **Pennsylvania:** Koop Community Health Information Center (College of Physicians of Philadelphia), **http://www.collphyphil.org/kooppg1.shtml**

- **Pennsylvania:** Learning Resources Center - Medical Library (Susquehanna Health System, Williamsport), **http://www.shscares.org/services/lrc/index.asp**

- **Pennsylvania:** Medical Library (UPMC Health System, Pittsburgh), **http://www.upmc.edu/passavant/library.htm**

- **Quebec, Canada:** Medical Library (Montreal General Hospital), **http://www.mghlib.mcgill.ca/**

- **South Dakota:** Rapid City Regional Hospital Medical Library (Rapid City Regional Hospital), **http://www.rcrh.org/Services/Library/Default.asp**

- **Texas:** Houston HealthWays (Houston Academy of Medicine-Texas Medical Center Library), **http://hhw.library.tmc.edu/**

- **Washington:** Community Health Library (Kittitas Valley Community Hospital), **http://www.kvch.com/**

- **Washington:** Southwest Washington Medical Center Library (Southwest Washington Medical Center, Vancouver), **http://www.swmedicalcenter.com/body.cfm?id=72**

ONLINE GLOSSARIES

The Internet provides access to a number of free-to-use medical dictionaries. The National Library of Medicine has compiled the following list of online dictionaries:

- ADAM Medical Encyclopedia (A.D.A.M., Inc.), comprehensive medical reference:
  http://www.nlm.nih.gov/medlineplus/encyclopedia.html

- MedicineNet.com Medical Dictionary (MedicineNet, Inc.):
  http://www.medterms.com/Script/Main/hp.asp

- Merriam-Webster Medical Dictionary (Inteli-Health, Inc.):
  http://www.intelihealth.com/IH/

- Multilingual Glossary of Technical and Popular Medical Terms in Eight European Languages (European Commission) - Danish, Dutch, English, French, German, Italian, Portuguese, and Spanish: **http://allserv.rug.ac.be/~rvdstich/eugloss/welcome.html**

- On-line Medical Dictionary (CancerWEB): **http://cancerweb.ncl.ac.uk/omd/**

- Rare Diseases Terms (Office of Rare Diseases):
  http://ord.aspensys.com/asp/diseases/diseases.asp

- Technology Glossary (National Library of Medicine) - Health Care Technology:
  http://www.nlm.nih.gov/nichsr/ta101/ta10108.htm

Beyond these, MEDLINEplus contains a very patient-friendly encyclopedia covering every aspect of medicine (licensed from A.D.A.M., Inc.). The ADAM Medical Encyclopedia can be accessed at **http://www.nlm.nih.gov/medlineplus/encyclopedia.html**. ADAM is also available on commercial Web sites such as drkoop.com (**http://www.drkoop.com/**) and Web MD (**http://my.webmd.com/adam/asset/adam_disease_articles/a_to_z/a**).

Online Dictionary Directories

The following are additional online directories compiled by the National Library of Medicine, including a number of specialized medical dictionaries:

- Medical Dictionaries: Medical & Biological (World Health Organization):
  http://www.who.int/hlt/virtuallibrary/English/diction.htm#Medical

- MEL-Michigan Electronic Library List of Online Health and Medical Dictionaries (Michigan Electronic Library): **http://mel.lib.mi.us/health/health-dictionaries.html**

- Patient Education: Glossaries (DMOZ Open Directory Project):
  http://dmoz.org/Health/Education/Patient_Education/Glossaries/

- Web of Online Dictionaries (Bucknell University):
  http://www.yourdictionary.com/diction5.html#medicine

AROMATHERAPY DICTIONARY

The definitions below are derived from official public sources, including the National Institutes of Health [NIH] and the European Union [EU].

Abdominal: Having to do with the abdomen, which is the part of the body between the chest and the hips that contains the pancreas, stomach, intestines, liver, gallbladder, and other organs. [NIH]

Abdominal Pain: Sensation of discomfort, distress, or agony in the abdominal region. [NIH]

Acceptor: A substance which, while normally not oxidized by oxygen or reduced by hydrogen, can be oxidized or reduced in presence of a substance which is itself undergoing oxidation or reduction. [NIH]

Accommodation: Adjustment, especially that of the eye for various distances. [EU]

Adrenal Cortex: The outer layer of the adrenal gland. It secretes mineralocorticoids, androgens, and glucocorticoids. [NIH]

Adverse Effect: An unwanted side effect of treatment. [NIH]

Alertness: A state of readiness to detect and respond to certain specified small changes occurring at random intervals in the environment. [NIH]

Algorithms: A procedure consisting of a sequence of algebraic formulas and/or logical steps to calculate or determine a given task. [NIH]

Alopecia: Absence of hair from areas where it is normally present. [NIH]

Alternative medicine: Practices not generally recognized by the medical community as standard or conventional medical approaches and used instead of standard treatments. Alternative medicine includes the taking of dietary supplements, megadose vitamins, and herbal preparations; the drinking of special teas; and practices such as massage therapy, magnet therapy, spiritual healing, and meditation. [NIH]

Amino Acids: Organic compounds that generally contain an amino (-NH2) and a carboxyl (-COOH) group. Twenty alpha-amino acids are the subunits which are polymerized to form proteins. [NIH]

Amino Acids: Organic compounds that generally contain an amino (-NH2) and a carboxyl (-COOH) group. Twenty alpha-amino acids are the subunits which are polymerized to form proteins. [NIH]

Analgesic: An agent that alleviates pain without causing loss of consciousness. [EU]

Antibody: A type of protein made by certain white blood cells in response to a foreign substance (antigen). Each antibody can bind to only a specific antigen. The purpose of this binding is to help destroy the antigen. Antibodies can work in several ways, depending on the nature of the antigen. Some antibodies destroy antigens directly. Others make it easier for white blood cells to destroy the antigen. [NIH]

Anti-inflammatory: Having to do with reducing inflammation. [NIH]

Anxiety: Persistent feeling of dread, apprehension, and impending disaster. [NIH]

Aqueous: Having to do with water. [NIH]

Aromatic: Having a spicy odour. [EU]

Arterial: Pertaining to an artery or to the arteries. [EU]

Arteries: The vessels carrying blood away from the heart. [NIH]

Autoimmune disease: A condition in which the body recognizes its own tissues as foreign and directs an immune response against them. [NIH]

Autopsy: Postmortem examination of the body. [NIH]

Base: In chemistry, the nonacid part of a salt; a substance that combines with acids to form salts; a substance that dissociates to give hydroxide ions in aqueous solutions; a substance whose molecule or ion can combine with a proton (hydrogen ion); a substance capable of donating a pair of electrons (to an acid) for the formation of a coordinate covalent bond. [EU]

Benign: Not cancerous; does not invade nearby tissue or spread to other parts of the body. [NIH]

Bereavement: Refers to the whole process of grieving and mourning and is associated with a deep sense of loss and sadness. [NIH]

Biotechnology: Body of knowledge related to the use of organisms, cells or cell-derived constituents for the purpose of developing products which are technically, scientifically and clinically useful. Alteration of biologic function at the molecular level (i.e., genetic engineering) is a central focus; laboratory methods used include transfection and cloning technologies, sequence and structure analysis algorithms, computer databases, and gene and protein structure function analysis and prediction. [NIH]

Bladder: The organ that stores urine. [NIH]

Bloating: Fullness or swelling in the abdomen that often occurs after meals. [NIH]

Blood pressure: The pressure of blood against the walls of a blood vessel or heart chamber. Unless there is reference to another location, such as the pulmonary artery or one of the heart chambers, it refers to the pressure in the systemic arteries, as measured, for example, in the forearm. [NIH]

Bone metastases: Cancer that has spread from the original (primary) tumor to the bone. [NIH]

Bone scan: A technique to create images of bones on a computer screen or on film. A small amount of radioactive material is injected into a blood vessel and travels through the bloodstream; it collects in the bones and is detected by a scanner. [NIH]

Bowel: The long tube-shaped organ in the abdomen that completes the process of digestion. There is both a small and a large bowel. Also called the intestine. [NIH]

Branch: Most commonly used for branches of nerves, but applied also to other structures. [NIH]

Bronchi: The larger air passages of the lungs arising from the terminal bifurcation of the trachea. [NIH]

Bronchitis: Inflammation (swelling and reddening) of the bronchi. [NIH]

Bullous: Pertaining to or characterized by bullae. [EU]

Burial: The act or ceremony of putting a corpse into the ground or a vault, or into the sea. The custom of burial is primeval and omnipresent in all cultures and civilizations, generally accompanied by ceremonial rites. [NIH]

Cardiovascular: Having to do with the heart and blood vessels. [NIH]

Cecum: The beginning of the large intestine. The cecum is connected to the lower part of the small intestine, called the ileum. [NIH]

Cell: The individual unit that makes up all of the tissues of the body. All living things are made up of one or more cells. [NIH]

Cell Division: The fission of a cell. [NIH]

Cellulose: A polysaccharide with glucose units linked as in cellobiose. It is the chief constituent of plant fibers, cotton being the purest natural form of the substance. As a raw material, it forms the basis for many derivatives used in chromatography, ion exchange materials, explosives manufacturing, and pharmaceutical preparations. [NIH]

Central Nervous System: The main information-processing organs of the nervous system, consisting of the brain, spinal cord, and meninges. [NIH]

Central Nervous System Infections: Pathogenic infections of the brain, spinal cord, and meninges. DNA virus infections; RNA virus infections; bacterial infections; mycoplasma infections; Spirochaetales infections; fungal infections; protozoan infections; helminthiasis; and prion diseases may involve the central nervous system as a primary or secondary process. [NIH]

Cerebral: Of or pertaining of the cerebrum or the brain. [EU]

Chamomile: Common name for several daisy-like species native to Europe and Western Asia, now naturalized in the United States and Australia. The dried flower-heads of two species, Anthemis nobilis (Chamaemelum nobile) and Matricaria recutita, have specific use as herbs. They are administered as tea, extracts, tinctures, or ointments. Chamomile contains choline, coumarins, cyanogenic glycosides, flavonoids, salicylate derivatives, tannins, and volatile oils. [NIH]

Character: In current usage, approximately equivalent to personality. The sum of the relatively fixed personality traits and habitual modes of response of an individual. [NIH]

Chiropractic: A system of treating bodily disorders by manipulation of the spine and other parts, based on the belief that the cause is the abnormal functioning of a nerve. [NIH]

Choline: A basic constituent of lecithin that is found in many plants and animal organs. It is important as a precursor of acetylcholine, as a methyl donor in various metabolic processes, and in lipid metabolism. [NIH]

Chronic: A disease or condition that persists or progresses over a long period of time. [NIH]

Chronic Disease: Disease or ailment of long duration. [NIH]

Clinical trial: A research study that tests how well new medical treatments or other interventions work in people. Each study is designed to test new methods of screening, prevention, diagnosis, or treatment of a disease. [NIH]

Cloning: The production of a number of genetically identical individuals; in genetic engineering, a process for the efficient replication of a great number of identical DNA molecules. [NIH]

Cofactor: A substance, microorganism or environmental factor that activates or enhances the action of another entity such as a disease-causing agent. [NIH]

Colitis: Inflammation of the colon. [NIH]

Color Therapy: A form of phototherapy using color to influence health and to treat various physical or mental disorders. The color rays may be in the visible or invisible spectrum and can be administered through colored lights or applied mentally through suggestion. [NIH]

Complement: A term originally used to refer to the heat-labile factor in serum that causes immune cytolysis, the lysis of antibody-coated cells, and now referring to the entire functionally related system comprising at least 20 distinct serum proteins that is the effector not only of immune cytolysis but also of other biologic functions. Complement activation occurs by two different sequences, the classic and alternative pathways. The proteins of the classic pathway are termed 'components of complement' and are designated by the symbols

C1 through C9. C1 is a calcium-dependent complex of three distinct proteins C1q, C1r and C1s. The proteins of the alternative pathway (collectively referred to as the properdin system) and complement regulatory proteins are known by semisystematic or trivial names. Fragments resulting from proteolytic cleavage of complement proteins are designated with lower-case letter suffixes, e.g., C3a. Inactivated fragments may be designated with the suffix 'i', e.g. C3bi. Activated components or complexes with biological activity are designated by a bar over the symbol e.g. C1 or C4b,2a. The classic pathway is activated by the binding of C1 to classic pathway activators, primarily antigen-antibody complexes containing IgM, IgG1, IgG3; C1q binds to a single IgM molecule or two adjacent IgG molecules. The alternative pathway can be activated by IgA immune complexes and also by nonimmunologic materials including bacterial endotoxins, microbial polysaccharides, and cell walls. Activation of the classic pathway triggers an enzymatic cascade involving C1, C4, C2 and C3; activation of the alternative pathway triggers a cascade involving C3 and factors B, D and P. Both result in the cleavage of C5 and the formation of the membrane attack complex. Complement activation also results in the formation of many biologically active complement fragments that act as anaphylatoxins, opsonins, or chemotactic factors. [EU]

Complementary and alternative medicine: CAM. Forms of treatment that are used in addition to (complementary) or instead of (alternative) standard treatments. These practices are not considered standard medical approaches. CAM includes dietary supplements, megadose vitamins, herbal preparations, special teas, massage therapy, magnet therapy, spiritual healing, and meditation. [NIH]

Complementary medicine: Practices not generally recognized by the medical community as standard or conventional medical approaches and used to enhance or complement the standard treatments. Complementary medicine includes the taking of dietary supplements, megadose vitamins, and herbal preparations; the drinking of special teas; and practices such as massage therapy, magnet therapy, spiritual healing, and meditation. [NIH]

Computational Biology: A field of biology concerned with the development of techniques for the collection and manipulation of biological data, and the use of such data to make biological discoveries or predictions. This field encompasses all computational methods and theories applicable to molecular biology and areas of computer-based techniques for solving biological problems including manipulation of models and datasets. [NIH]

Computed tomography: CT scan. A series of detailed pictures of areas inside the body, taken from different angles; the pictures are created by a computer linked to an x-ray machine. Also called computerized tomography and computerized axial tomography (CAT) scan. [NIH]

Computerized axial tomography: A series of detailed pictures of areas inside the body, taken from different angles; the pictures are created by a computer linked to an x-ray machine. Also called CAT scan, computed tomography (CT scan), or computerized tomography. [NIH]

Conception: The onset of pregnancy, marked by implantation of the blastocyst; the formation of a viable zygote. [EU]

Cone: One of the special retinal receptor elements which are presumed to be primarily concerned with perception of light and color stimuli when the eye is adapted to light. [NIH]

Consciousness: Sense of awareness of self and of the environment. [NIH]

Constipation: Infrequent or difficult evacuation of feces. [NIH]

Contact dermatitis: Inflammation of the skin with varying degrees of erythema, edema and vesinculation resulting from cutaneous contact with a foreign substance or other exposure. [NIH]

Contraindications: Any factor or sign that it is unwise to pursue a certain kind of action or treatment, e. g. giving a general anesthetic to a person with pneumonia. [NIH]

Coordination: Muscular or motor regulation or the harmonious cooperation of muscles or groups of muscles, in a complex action or series of actions. [NIH]

Coronary: Encircling in the manner of a crown; a term applied to vessels; nerves, ligaments, etc. The term usually denotes the arteries that supply the heart muscle and, by extension, a pathologic involvement of them. [EU]

Coronary Thrombosis: Presence of a thrombus in a coronary artery, often causing a myocardial infarction. [NIH]

Corpus: The body of the uterus. [NIH]

Corpus Luteum: The yellow glandular mass formed in the ovary by an ovarian follicle that has ruptured and discharged its ovum. [NIH]

Coumarins: Synthetic or naturally occurring substances related to coumarin, the delta-lactone of coumarinic acid. Coumarin itself occurs in the tonka bean. The various coumarins have a wide range of proposed actions and uses including as anticoagulants, pharmaceutical aids, indicators and reagents, photoreactive substances, and antineoplastic agents. [NIH]

Cranial: Pertaining to the cranium, or to the anterior (in animals) or superior (in humans) end of the body. [EU]

Craniocerebral Trauma: Traumatic injuries involving the cranium and intracranial structures (i.e., brain; cranial nerves; meninges; and other structures). Injuries may be classified by whether or not the skull is penetrated (i.e., penetrating vs. nonpenetrating) or whether there is an associated hemorrhage. [NIH]

Curative: Tending to overcome disease and promote recovery. [EU]

Curettage: Removal of tissue with a curette, a spoon-shaped instrument with a sharp edge. [NIH]

Curette: A spoon-shaped instrument with a sharp edge. [NIH]

Cutaneous: Having to do with the skin. [NIH]

Cytotoxic: Cell-killing. [NIH]

Databases, Bibliographic: Extensive collections, reputedly complete, of references and citations to books, articles, publications, etc., generally on a single subject or specialized subject area. Databases can operate through automated files, libraries, or computer disks. The concept should be differentiated from factual databases which is used for collections of data and facts apart from bibliographic references to them. [NIH]

Death, Sudden: The sudden cessation of all vital bodily functions, manifested by the permanent loss of total cerebral, respiratory, and cardiovascular functions. [NIH]

Degenerative: Undergoing degeneration : tending to degenerate; having the character of or involving degeneration; causing or tending to cause degeneration. [EU]

Dementia: An acquired organic mental disorder with loss of intellectual abilities of sufficient severity to interfere with social or occupational functioning. The dysfunction is multifaceted and involves memory, behavior, personality, judgment, attention, spatial relations, language, abstract thought, and other executive functions. The intellectual decline is usually progressive, and initially spares the level of consciousness. [NIH]

Dermatitis: Any inflammation of the skin. [NIH]

Dermatology: A medical specialty concerned with the skin, its structure, functions, diseases, and treatment. [NIH]

Diagnostic procedure: A method used to identify a disease. [NIH]

Dialyzer: A part of the hemodialysis machine. (See hemodialysis under dialysis.) The dialyzer has two sections separated by a membrane. One section holds dialysate. The other holds the patient's blood. [NIH]

Diarrhea: Passage of excessively liquid or excessively frequent stools. [NIH]

Digestion: The process of breakdown of food for metabolism and use by the body. [NIH]

Digestive system: The organs that take in food and turn it into products that the body can use to stay healthy. Waste products the body cannot use leave the body through bowel movements. The digestive system includes the salivary glands, mouth, esophagus, stomach, liver, pancreas, gallbladder, small and large intestines, and rectum. [NIH]

Digestive tract: The organs through which food passes when food is eaten. These organs are the mouth, esophagus, stomach, small and large intestines, and rectum. [NIH]

Diploid: Having two sets of chromosomes. [NIH]

Direct: 1. Straight; in a straight line. 2. Performed immediately and without the intervention of subsidiary means. [EU]

Disease Vectors: Invertebrates or non-human vertebrates which transmit infective organisms from one host to another. [NIH]

Disinfectant: An agent that disinfects; applied particularly to agents used on inanimate objects. [EU]

Dispenser: Glass, metal or plastic shell fitted with valve from which a pressurized formulation is dispensed; an instrument for atomizing. [NIH]

Dissociation: 1. The act of separating or state of being separated. 2. The separation of a molecule into two or more fragments (atoms, molecules, ions, or free radicals) produced by the absorption of light or thermal energy or by solvation. 3. In psychology, a defense mechanism in which a group of mental processes are segregated from the rest of a person's mental activity in order to avoid emotional distress, as in the dissociative disorders (q.v.), or in which an idea or object is segregated from its emotional significance; in the first sense it is roughly equivalent to splitting, in the second, to isolation. 4. A defect of mental integration in which one or more groups of mental processes become separated off from normal consciousness and, thus separated, function as a unitary whole. [EU]

Drug Interactions: The action of a drug that may affect the activity, metabolism, or toxicity of another drug. [NIH]

Dyes: Chemical substances that are used to stain and color other materials. The coloring may or may not be permanent. Dyes can also be used as therapeutic agents and test reagents in medicine and scientific research. [NIH]

Edema: Excessive amount of watery fluid accumulated in the intercellular spaces, most commonly present in subcutaneous tissue. [NIH]

Electrons: Stable elementary particles having the smallest known negative charge, present in all elements; also called negatrons. Positively charged electrons are called positrons. The numbers, energies and arrangement of electrons around atomic nuclei determine the chemical identities of elements. Beams of electrons are called cathode rays or beta rays, the latter being a high-energy biproduct of nuclear decay. [NIH]

Embryo: The prenatal stage of mammalian development characterized by rapid morphological changes and the differentiation of basic structures. [NIH]

Emollient: Softening or soothing; called also malactic. [EU]

Energetic: Exhibiting energy : strenuous; operating with force, vigour, or effect. [EU]

Environmental Health: The science of controlling or modifying those conditions, influences, or forces surrounding man which relate to promoting, establishing, and maintaining health. [NIH]

Environmental Medicine: Medical specialty concerned with environmental factors that may impinge upon human disease, and development of methods for the detection, prevention, and control of environmentally related disease. [NIH]

Enzyme: A protein that speeds up chemical reactions in the body. [NIH]

Erythema: Redness of the skin produced by congestion of the capillaries. This condition may result from a variety of causes. [NIH]

Esophagus: The muscular tube through which food passes from the throat to the stomach. [NIH]

Estrogen: One of the two female sex hormones. [NIH]

Evacuation: An emptying, as of the bowels. [EU]

Extensor: A muscle whose contraction tends to straighten a limb; the antagonist of a flexor. [NIH]

Family Planning: Programs or services designed to assist the family in controlling reproduction by either improving or diminishing fertility. [NIH]

Fat: Total lipids including phospholipids. [NIH]

Feces: The excrement discharged from the intestines, consisting of bacteria, cells exfoliated from the intestines, secretions, chiefly of the liver, and a small amount of food residue. [EU]

Fetus: The developing offspring from 7 to 8 weeks after conception until birth. [NIH]

Fleas: Parasitic, blood-sucking, wingless insects comprising the order Siphonaptera. [NIH]

Fold: A plication or doubling of various parts of the body. [NIH]

Fraud: Exploitation through misrepresentation of the facts or concealment of the purposes of the exploiter. [NIH]

Freeze Drying: Method of tissue preparation in which the tissue specimen is frozen and then dehydrated at low temperature in a high vacuum. This method is also used for dehydrating pharmaceutical and food products. [NIH]

Frontal Lobe: The anterior part of the cerebral hemisphere. [NIH]

Gamma Rays: Very powerful and penetrating, high-energy electromagnetic radiation of shorter wavelength than that of x-rays. They are emitted by a decaying nucleus, usually between 0.01 and 10 MeV. They are also called nuclear x-rays. [NIH]

Gas: Air that comes from normal breakdown of food. The gases are passed out of the body through the rectum (flatus) or the mouth (burp). [NIH]

Gastroenterologist: A doctor who specializes in diagnosing and treating disorders of the digestive system. [NIH]

Gastrointestinal: Refers to the stomach and intestines. [NIH]

Gastrointestinal tract: The stomach and intestines. [NIH]

Gels: Colloids with a solid continuous phase and liquid as the dispersed phase; gels may be unstable when, due to temperature or other cause, the solid phase liquifies; the resulting colloid is called a sol. [NIH]

Gene: The functional and physical unit of heredity passed from parent to offspring. Genes are pieces of DNA, and most genes contain the information for making a specific protein. [NIH]

Geriatric: Pertaining to the treatment of the aged. [EU]

Gestation: The period of development of the young in viviparous animals, from the time of fertilization of the ovum until birth. [EU]

Governing Board: The group in which legal authority is vested for the control of health-related institutions and organizations. [NIH]

Growth: The progressive development of a living being or part of an organism from its earliest stage to maturity. [NIH]

Habitual: Of the nature of a habit; according to habit; established by or repeated by force of habit, customary. [EU]

Haploid: An organism with one basic chromosome set, symbolized by n; the normal condition of gametes in diploids. [NIH]

Headache: Pain in the cranial region that may occur as an isolated and benign symptom or as a manifestation of a wide variety of conditions including subarachnoid hemorrhage; craniocerebral trauma; central nervous system infections; intracranial hypertension; and other disorders. In general, recurrent headaches that are not associated with a primary disease process are referred to as headache disorders (e.g., migraine). [NIH]

Headache Disorders: Common conditions characterized by persistent or recurrent headaches. Headache syndrome classification systems may be based on etiology (e.g., vascular headache, post-traumatic headaches, etc.), temporal pattern (e.g., cluster headache, paroxysmal hemicrania, etc.), and precipitating factors (e.g., cough headache). [NIH]

Hemodialysis: The use of a machine to clean wastes from the blood after the kidneys have failed. The blood travels through tubes to a dialyzer, which removes wastes and extra fluid. The cleaned blood then flows through another set of tubes back into the body. [NIH]

Hemorrhage: Bleeding or escape of blood from a vessel. [NIH]

Hepatitis: Inflammation of the liver and liver disease involving degenerative or necrotic alterations of hepatocytes. [NIH]

Hepatocytes: The main structural component of the liver. They are specialized epithelial cells that are organized into interconnected plates called lobules. [NIH]

Heredity: 1. The genetic transmission of a particular quality or trait from parent to offspring. 2. The genetic constitution of an individual. [EU]

Histology: The study of tissues and cells under a microscope. [NIH]

Hormonal: Pertaining to or of the nature of a hormone. [EU]

Hormone: A substance in the body that regulates certain organs. Hormones such as gastrin help in breaking down food. Some hormones come from cells in the stomach and small intestine. [NIH]

Hospice: Institution dedicated to caring for the terminally ill. [NIH]

Hydrogen: The first chemical element in the periodic table. It has the atomic symbol H, atomic number 1, and atomic weight 1. It exists, under normal conditions, as a colorless, odorless, tasteless, diatomic gas. Hydrogen ions are protons. Besides the common H1 isotope, hydrogen exists as the stable isotope deuterium and the unstable, radioactive isotope tritium. [NIH]

Hypertension: Persistently high arterial blood pressure. Currently accepted threshold levels are 140 mm Hg systolic and 90 mm Hg diastolic pressure. [NIH]

Hypnotherapy: Sleeping-cure. [NIH]

Id: The part of the personality structure which harbors the unconscious instinctive desires and strivings of the individual. [NIH]

Immune response: The activity of the immune system against foreign substances (antigens). [NIH]

Immune system: The organs, cells, and molecules responsible for the recognition and disposal of foreign ("non-self") material which enters the body. [NIH]

Immunodeficiency: The decreased ability of the body to fight infection and disease. [NIH]

Immunologic: The ability of the antibody-forming system to recall a previous experience with an antigen and to respond to a second exposure with the prompt production of large amounts of antibody. [NIH]

Indicative: That indicates; that points out more or less exactly; that reveals fairly clearly. [EU]

Infarction: A pathological process consisting of a sudden insufficient blood supply to an area, which results in necrosis of that area. It is usually caused by a thrombus, an embolus, or a vascular torsion. [NIH]

Infection: 1. Invasion and multiplication of microorganisms in body tissues, which may be clinically unapparent or result in local cellular injury due to competitive metabolism, toxins, intracellular replication, or antigen-antibody response. The infection may remain localized, subclinical, and temporary if the body's defensive mechanisms are effective. A local infection may persist and spread by extension to become an acute, subacute, or chronic clinical infection or disease state. A local infection may also become systemic when the microorganisms gain access to the lymphatic or vascular system. 2. An infectious disease. [EU]

Inflammation: A pathological process characterized by injury or destruction of tissues caused by a variety of cytologic and chemical reactions. It is usually manifested by typical signs of pain, heat, redness, swelling, and loss of function. [NIH]

Inflammatory bowel disease: A general term that refers to the inflammation of the colon and rectum. Inflammatory bowel disease includes ulcerative colitis and Crohn's disease. [NIH]

Inhalation: The drawing of air or other substances into the lungs. [EU]

Insecticides: Pesticides designed to control insects that are harmful to man. The insects may be directly harmful, as those acting as disease vectors, or indirectly harmful, as destroyers of crops, food products, or textile fabrics. [NIH]

Insomnia: Difficulty in going to sleep or getting enough sleep. [NIH]

Insulator: Material covering the metal conductor of the lead. It is usually polyurethane or silicone. [NIH]

Intensive Care: Advanced and highly specialized care provided to medical or surgical patients whose conditions are life-threatening and require comprehensive care and constant monitoring. It is usually administered in specially equipped units of a health care facility. [NIH]

Intermittent: Occurring at separated intervals; having periods of cessation of activity. [EU]

Intestine: A long, tube-shaped organ in the abdomen that completes the process of digestion. There is both a large intestine and a small intestine. Also called the bowel. [NIH]

Involuntary: Reaction occurring without intention or volition. [NIH]

Ionization: 1. Any process by which a neutral atom gains or loses electrons, thus acquiring a net charge, as the dissociation of a substance in solution into ions or ion production by the passage of radioactive particles. 2. Iontophoresis. [EU]

Ionizing: Radiation comprising charged particles, e. g. electrons, protons, alpha-particles, etc., having sufficient kinetic energy to produce ionization by collision. [NIH]

Ions: An atom or group of atoms that have a positive or negative electric charge due to a gain (negative charge) or loss (positive charge) of one or more electrons. Atoms with a positive charge are known as cations; those with a negative charge are anions. [NIH]

Irritable Bowel Syndrome: A disorder that comes and goes. Nerves that control the muscles in the GI tract are too active. The GI tract becomes sensitive to food, stool, gas, and stress. Causes abdominal pain, bloating, and constipation or diarrhea. Also called spastic colon or mucous colitis. [NIH]

Jealousy: An irrational reaction compounded of grief, loss of self-esteem, enmity against the rival and self criticism. [NIH]

Joint: The point of contact between elements of an animal skeleton with the parts that surround and support it. [NIH]

Kb: A measure of the length of DNA fragments, 1 Kb = 1000 base pairs. The largest DNA fragments are up to 50 kilobases long. [NIH]

Keratin: A class of fibrous proteins or scleroproteins important both as structural proteins and as keys to the study of protein conformation. The family represents the principal constituent of epidermis, hair, nails, horny tissues, and the organic matrix of tooth enamel. Two major conformational groups have been characterized, alpha-keratin, whose peptide backbone forms an alpha-helix, and beta-keratin, whose backbone forms a zigzag or pleated sheet structure. [NIH]

Kinetic: Pertaining to or producing motion. [EU]

Large Intestine: The part of the intestine that goes from the cecum to the rectum. The large intestine absorbs water from stool and changes it from a liquid to a solid form. The large intestine is 5 feet long and includes the appendix, cecum, colon, and rectum. Also called colon. [NIH]

Lens: The transparent, double convex (outward curve on both sides) structure suspended between the aqueous and vitreous; helps to focus light on the retina. [NIH]

Leucocyte: All the white cells of the blood and their precursors (myeloid cell series, lymphoid cell series) but commonly used to indicate granulocytes exclusive of lymphocytes. [NIH]

Leukaemia: An acute or chronic disease of unknown cause in man and other warm-blooded animals that involves the blood-forming organs, is characterized by an abnormal increase in the number of leucocytes in the tissues of the body with or without a corresponding increase of those in the circulating blood, and is classified according of the type leucocyte most prominently involved. [EU]

Library Services: Services offered to the library user. They include reference and circulation. [NIH]

Life cycle: The successive stages through which an organism passes from fertilized ovum or spore to the fertilized ovum or spore of the next generation. [NIH]

Lipid: Fat. [NIH]

Liver: A large, glandular organ located in the upper abdomen. The liver cleanses the blood and aids in digestion by secreting bile. [NIH]

Liver scan: An image of the liver created on a computer screen or on film. A radioactive substance is injected into a blood vessel and travels through the bloodstream. It collects in the liver, especially in abnormal areas, and can be detected by the scanner. [NIH]

Localized: Cancer which has not metastasized yet. [NIH]

Locomotion: Movement or the ability to move from one place or another. It can refer to humans, vertebrate or invertebrate animals, and microorganisms. [NIH]

Magnetic Resonance Imaging: Non-invasive method of demonstrating internal anatomy based on the principle that atomic nuclei in a strong magnetic field absorb pulses of radiofrequency energy and emit them as radiowaves which can be reconstructed into computerized images. The concept includes proton spin tomographic techniques. [NIH]

Malignant: Cancerous; a growth with a tendency to invade and destroy nearby tissue and spread to other parts of the body. [NIH]

MEDLINE: An online database of MEDLARS, the computerized bibliographic Medical Literature Analysis and Retrieval System of the National Library of Medicine. [NIH]

Membranes: Thin layers of tissue which cover parts of the body, separate adjacent cavities, or connect adjacent structures. [NIH]

Memory: Complex mental function having four distinct phases: (1) memorizing or learning, (2) retention, (3) recall, and (4) recognition. Clinically, it is usually subdivided into immediate, recent, and remote memory. [NIH]

Menstrual Cycle: The period of the regularly recurring physiologic changes in the endometrium occurring during the reproductive period in human females and some primates and culminating in partial sloughing of the endometrium (menstruation). [NIH]

Menstruation: The normal physiologic discharge through the vagina of blood and mucosal tissues from the nonpregnant uterus. [NIH]

Mental Disorders: Psychiatric illness or diseases manifested by breakdowns in the adaptational process expressed primarily as abnormalities of thought, feeling, and behavior producing either distress or impairment of function. [NIH]

Mental Health: The state wherein the person is well adjusted. [NIH]

MI: Myocardial infarction. Gross necrosis of the myocardium as a result of interruption of the blood supply to the area; it is almost always caused by atherosclerosis of the coronary arteries, upon which coronary thrombosis is usually superimposed. [NIH]

Midwifery: The practice of assisting women in childbirth. [NIH]

Milliliter: A measure of volume for a liquid. A milliliter is approximately 950-times smaller than a quart and 30-times smaller than a fluid ounce. A milliliter of liquid and a cubic centimeter (cc) of liquid are the same. [NIH]

Miscarriage: Spontaneous expulsion of the products of pregnancy before the middle of the second trimester. [NIH]

Molecular: Of, pertaining to, or composed of molecules : a very small mass of matter. [EU]

Molecule: A chemical made up of two or more atoms. The atoms in a molecule can be the same (an oxygen molecule has two oxygen atoms) or different (a water molecule has two hydrogen atoms and one oxygen atom). Biological molecules, such as proteins and DNA, can be made up of many thousands of atoms. [NIH]

Monitor: An apparatus which automatically records such physiological signs as respiration, pulse, and blood pressure in an anesthetized patient or one undergoing surgical or other procedures. [NIH]

Morphological: Relating to the configuration or the structure of live organs. [NIH]

Mucosa: A mucous membrane, or tunica mucosa. [EU]

Mucus: The viscous secretion of mucous membranes. It contains mucin, white blood cells, water, inorganic salts, and exfoliated cells. [NIH]

Multiple sclerosis: A disorder of the central nervous system marked by weakness, numbness, a loss of muscle coordination, and problems with vision, speech, and bladder control. Multiple sclerosis is thought to be an autoimmune disease in which the body's immune system destroys myelin. Myelin is a substance that contains both protein and fat (lipid) and serves as a nerve insulator and helps in the transmission of nerve signals. [NIH]

Myelin: The fatty substance that covers and protects nerves. [NIH]

Myocardium: The muscle tissue of the heart composed of striated, involuntary muscle known as cardiac muscle. [NIH]

Nasal Cavity: The proximal portion of the respiratory passages on either side of the nasal septum, lined with ciliated mucosa, extending from the nares to the pharynx. [NIH]

Nasal Septum: The partition separating the two nasal cavities in the midplane, composed of cartilaginous, membranous and bony parts. [NIH]

Nausea: An unpleasant sensation in the stomach usually accompanied by the urge to vomit. Common causes are early pregnancy, sea and motion sickness, emotional stress, intense pain, food poisoning, and various enteroviruses. [NIH]

Necrosis: A pathological process caused by the progressive degradative action of enzymes that is generally associated with severe cellular trauma. It is characterized by mitochondrial swelling, nuclear flocculation, uncontrolled cell lysis, and ultimately cell death. [NIH]

Need: A state of tension or dissatisfaction felt by an individual that impels him to action toward a goal he believes will satisfy the impulse. [NIH]

Neonatal: Pertaining to the first four weeks after birth. [EU]

Neoplasms: New abnormal growth of tissue. Malignant neoplasms show a greater degree of anaplasia and have the properties of invasion and metastasis, compared to benign neoplasms. [NIH]

Nerve: A cordlike structure of nervous tissue that connects parts of the nervous system with other tissues of the body and conveys nervous impulses to, or away from, these tissues. [NIH]

Nervous System: The entire nerve apparatus composed of the brain, spinal cord, nerves and ganglia. [NIH]

Nonverbal Communication: Transmission of emotions, ideas, and attitudes between individuals in ways other than the spoken language. [NIH]

Nursing Care: Care given to patients by nursing service personnel. [NIH]

Observational study: An epidemiologic study that does not involve any intervention, experimental or otherwise. Such a study may be one in which nature is allowed to take its course, with changes in one characteristic being studied in relation to changes in other characteristics. Analytical epidemiologic methods, such as case-control and cohort study designs, are properly called observational epidemiology because the investigator is observing without intervention other than to record, classify, count, and statistically analyze results. [NIH]

Odour: A volatile emanation that is perceived by the sense of smell. [EU]

Ointments: Semisolid preparations used topically for protective emollient effects or as a vehicle for local administration of medications. Ointment bases are various mixtures of fats, waxes, animal and plant oils and solid and liquid hydrocarbons. [NIH]

Ovum: A female germ cell extruded from the ovary at ovulation. [NIH]

Oxidation: The act of oxidizing or state of being oxidized. Chemically it consists in the increase of positive charges on an atom or the loss of negative charges. Most biological oxidations are accomplished by the removal of a pair of hydrogen atoms (dehydrogenation) from a molecule. Such oxidations must be accompanied by reduction of an acceptor molecule. Univalent o. indicates loss of one electron; divalent o., the loss of two electrons. [EU]

Palliative: 1. Affording relief, but not cure. 2. An alleviating medicine. [EU]

Paraffin: A mixture of solid hydrocarbons obtained from petroleum It has a wide range of uses including as a stiffening agent in ointments, as a lubricant, and as a topical anti-inflammatory. It is also commonly used as an embedding material in histology. [NIH]

Pathologic: 1. Indicative of or caused by a morbid condition. 2. Pertaining to pathology (= branch of medicine that treats the essential nature of the disease, especially the structural and functional changes in tissues and organs of the body caused by the disease). [EU]

Patient Education: The teaching or training of patients concerning their own health needs. [NIH]

Perception: The ability quickly and accurately to recognize similarities and differences among presented objects, whether these be pairs of words, pairs of number series, or multiple sets of these or other symbols such as geometric figures. [NIH]

Perinatal: Pertaining to or occurring in the period shortly before and after birth; variously defined as beginning with completion of the twentieth to twenty-eighth week of gestation and ending 7 to 28 days after birth. [EU]

Petroleum: Naturally occurring complex liquid hydrocarbons which, after distillation, yield combustible fuels, petrochemicals, and lubricants. [NIH]

Pharmacologic: Pertaining to pharmacology or to the properties and reactions of drugs. [EU]

Pharynx: The hollow tube about 5 inches long that starts behind the nose and ends at the top of the trachea (windpipe) and esophagus (the tube that goes to the stomach). [NIH]

Phospholipids: Lipids containing one or more phosphate groups, particularly those derived from either glycerol (phosphoglycerides; glycerophospholipids) or sphingosine (sphingolipids). They are polar lipids that are of great importance for the structure and function of cell membranes and are the most abundant of membrane lipids, although not stored in large amounts in the system. [NIH]

Phototherapy: Treatment of disease by exposure to light, especially by variously concentrated light rays or specific wavelengths. [NIH]

Pilot study: The initial study examining a new method or treatment. [NIH]

Placenta: A highly vascular fetal organ through which the fetus absorbs oxygen and other nutrients and excretes carbon dioxide and other wastes. It begins to form about the eighth day of gestation when the blastocyst adheres to the decidua. [NIH]

Plants: Multicellular, eukaryotic life forms of the kingdom Plantae. They are characterized by a mainly photosynthetic mode of nutrition; essentially unlimited growth at localized regions of cell divisions (meristems); cellulose within cells providing rigidity; the absence of organs of locomotion; absense of nervous and sensory systems; and an alteration of haploid and diploid generations. [NIH]

Practice Guidelines: Directions or principles presenting current or future rules of policy for the health care practitioner to assist him in patient care decisions regarding diagnosis, therapy, or related clinical circumstances. The guidelines may be developed by government agencies at any level, institutions, professional societies, governing boards, or by the convening of expert panels. The guidelines form a basis for the evaluation of all aspects of health care and delivery. [NIH]

Premenstrual: Occurring before menstruation. [EU]

Premenstrual Syndrome: A syndrome occurring most often during the last week of the menstrual cycle and ending soon after the onset of menses. Some of the symptoms are emotional instability, insomnia, headache, nausea, vomiting, abdominal distension, and painful breasts. [NIH]

Prenatal: Existing or occurring before birth, with reference to the fetus. [EU]

Progesterone: Pregn-4-ene-3,20-dione. The principal progestational hormone of the body, secreted by the corpus luteum, adrenal cortex, and placenta. Its chief function is to prepare the uterus for the reception and development of the fertilized ovum. It acts as an antiovulatory agent when administered on days 5-25 of the menstrual cycle. [NIH]

Progressive: Advancing; going forward; going from bad to worse; increasing in scope or severity. [EU]

Protein S: The vitamin K-dependent cofactor of activated protein C. Together with protein C, it inhibits the action of factors VIIIa and Va. A deficiency in protein S can lead to recurrent venous and arterial thrombosis. [NIH]

Proteins: Polymers of amino acids linked by peptide bonds. The specific sequence of amino acids determines the shape and function of the protein. [NIH]

Protons: Stable elementary particles having the smallest known positive charge, found in the nuclei of all elements. The proton mass is less than that of a neutron. A proton is the nucleus of the light hydrogen atom, i.e., the hydrogen ion. [NIH]

Proximal: Nearest; closer to any point of reference; opposed to distal. [EU]

Pruritus: An intense itching sensation that produces the urge to rub or scratch the skin to obtain relief. [NIH]

Psoriasis: A common genetically determined, chronic, inflammatory skin disease characterized by rounded erythematous, dry, scaling patches. The lesions have a predilection for nails, scalp, genitalia, extensor surfaces, and the lumbosacral region. Accelerated epidermopoiesis is considered to be the fundamental pathologic feature in psoriasis. [NIH]

Psychoneuroimmunology: The field concerned with the interrelationship between the brain, behavior and the immune system. Neuropsychologic, neuroanatomic and psychosocial studies have demonstrated their role in accentuating or diminishing immune/allergic responses. [NIH]

Psychotherapy: A generic term for the treatment of mental illness or emotional disturbances primarily by verbal or nonverbal communication. [NIH]

Public Policy: A course or method of action selected, usually by a government, from among alternatives to guide and determine present and future decisions. [NIH]

Pulmonary: Relating to the lungs. [NIH]

Pulse: The rhythmical expansion and contraction of an artery produced by waves of pressure caused by the ejection of blood from the left ventricle of the heart as it contracts. [NIH]

Race: A population within a species which exhibits general similarities within itself, but is both discontinuous and distinct from other populations of that species, though not sufficiently so as to achieve the status of a taxon. [NIH]

Radiation: Emission or propagation of electromagnetic energy (waves/rays), or the waves/rays themselves; a stream of electromagnetic particles (electrons, neutrons, protons, alpha particles) or a mixture of these. The most common source is the sun. [NIH]

Radioactive: Giving off radiation. [NIH]

Radioimmunotherapy: Radiotherapy where cytotoxic radionuclides are linked to antibodies in order to deliver toxins directly to tumor targets. Therapy with targeted radiation rather than antibody-targeted toxins (immunotoxins) has the advantage that adjacent tumor cells, which lack the appropriate antigenic determinants, can be destroyed by radiation cross-fire.

Radioimmunotherapy is sometimes called targeted radiotherapy, but this latter term can also refer to radionuclides linked to non-immune molecules (radiotherapy). [NIH]

Radiotherapy: The use of ionizing radiation to treat malignant neoplasms and other benign conditions. The most common forms of ionizing radiation used as therapy are x-rays, gamma rays, and electrons. A special form of radiotherapy, targeted radiotherapy, links a cytotoxic radionuclide to a molecule that targets the tumor. When this molecule is an antibody or other immunologic molecule, the technique is called radioimmunotherapy. [NIH]

Randomized: Describes an experiment or clinical trial in which animal or human subjects are assigned by chance to separate groups that compare different treatments. [NIH]

Receptor: A molecule inside or on the surface of a cell that binds to a specific substance and causes a specific physiologic effect in the cell. [NIH]

Rectum: The last 8 to 10 inches of the large intestine. [NIH]

Refer: To send or direct for treatment, aid, information, de decision. [NIH]

Reflex: An involuntary movement or exercise of function in a part, excited in response to a stimulus applied to the periphery and transmitted to the brain or spinal cord. [NIH]

Respiration: The act of breathing with the lungs, consisting of inspiration, or the taking into the lungs of the ambient air, and of expiration, or the expelling of the modified air which contains more carbon dioxide than the air taken in (Blakiston's Gould Medical Dictionary, 4th ed.). This does not include tissue respiration (= oxygen consumption) or cell respiration (= cell respiration). [NIH]

Retina: The ten-layered nervous tissue membrane of the eye. It is continuous with the optic nerve and receives images of external objects and transmits visual impulses to the brain. Its outer surface is in contact with the choroid and the inner surface with the vitreous body. The outer-most layer is pigmented, whereas the inner nine layers are transparent. [NIH]

Retinal: 1. Pertaining to the retina. 2. The aldehyde of retinol, derived by the oxidative enzymatic splitting of absorbed dietary carotene, and having vitamin A activity. In the retina, retinal combines with opsins to form visual pigments. One isomer, 11-cis retinal combines with opsin in the rods (scotopsin) to form rhodopsin, or visual purple. Another, all-trans retinal (trans-r.); visual yellow; xanthopsin) results from the bleaching of rhodopsin by light, in which the 11-cis form is converted to the all-trans form. Retinal also combines with opsins in the cones (photopsins) to form the three pigments responsible for colour vision. Called also retinal, and retinene1. [EU]

Retinoids: Derivatives of vitamin A. Used dinically in the treatment of severe cystic acne, psoriasis, and other disorders of keratinization. Their possible use in the prophylaxis and treatment of cancer is being actively explored. [NIH]

Rigidity: Stiffness or inflexibility, chiefly that which is abnormal or morbid; rigor. [EU]

Salicylate: Non-steroidal anti-inflammatory drugs. [NIH]

Scans: Pictures of structures inside the body. Scans often used in diagnosing, staging, and monitoring disease include liver scans, bone scans, and computed tomography (CT) or computerized axial tomography (CAT) scans and magnetic resonance imaging (MRI) scans. In liver scanning and bone scanning, radioactive substances that are injected into the bloodstream collect in these organs. A scanner that detects the radiation is used to create pictures. In CT scanning, an x-ray machine linked to a computer is used to produce detailed pictures of organs inside the body. MRI scans use a large magnet connected to a computer to create pictures of areas inside the body. [NIH]

Sclerosis: A pathological process consisting of hardening or fibrosis of an anatomical structure, often a vessel or a nerve. [NIH]

Screening: Checking for disease when there are no symptoms. [NIH]

Sebaceous: Gland that secretes sebum. [NIH]

Sebaceous gland: Gland that secretes sebum. [NIH]

Sebum: The oily substance secreted by sebaceous glands. It is composed of keratin, fat, and cellular debris. [NIH]

Sedative: 1. Allaying activity and excitement. 2. An agent that allays excitement. [EU]

Shock: The general bodily disturbance following a severe injury; an emotional or moral upset occasioned by some disturbing or unexpected experience; disruption of the circulation, which can upset all body functions: sometimes referred to as circulatory shock. [NIH]

Side effect: A consequence other than the one(s) for which an agent or measure is used, as the adverse effects produced by a drug, especially on a tissue or organ system other than the one sought to be benefited by its administration. [EU]

Skeleton: The framework that supports the soft tissues of vertebrate animals and protects many of their internal organs. The skeletons of vertebrates are made of bone and/or cartilage. [NIH]

Small intestine: The part of the digestive tract that is located between the stomach and the large intestine. [NIH]

Solvent: 1. Dissolving; effecting a solution. 2. A liquid that dissolves or that is capable of dissolving; the component of a solution that is present in greater amount. [EU]

Spastic: 1. Of the nature of or characterized by spasms. 2. Hypertonic, so that the muscles are stiff and the movements awkward. 3. A person exhibiting spasticity, such as occurs in spastic paralysis or in cerebral palsy. [EU]

Specialist: In medicine, one who concentrates on 1 special branch of medical science. [NIH]

Species: A taxonomic category subordinate to a genus (or subgenus) and superior to a subspecies or variety, composed of individuals possessing common characters distinguishing them from other categories of individuals of the same taxonomic level. In taxonomic nomenclature, species are designated by the genus name followed by a Latin or Latinized adjective or noun. [EU]

Spectrum: A charted band of wavelengths of electromagnetic vibrations obtained by refraction and diffraction. By extension, a measurable range of activity, such as the range of bacteria affected by an antibiotic (antibacterial s.) or the complete range of manifestations of a disease. [EU]

Spinal cord: The main trunk or bundle of nerves running down the spine through holes in the spinal bone (the vertebrae) from the brain to the level of the lower back. [NIH]

Staging: Performing exams and tests to learn the extent of the cancer within the body, especially whether the disease has spread from the original site to other parts of the body. [NIH]

Stillbirth: The birth of a dead fetus or baby. [NIH]

Stimulus: That which can elicit or evoke action (response) in a muscle, nerve, gland or other excitable issue, or cause an augmenting action upon any function or metabolic process. [NIH]

Stomach: An organ of digestion situated in the left upper quadrant of the abdomen between the termination of the esophagus and the beginning of the duodenum. [NIH]

Stool: The waste matter discharged in a bowel movement; feces. [NIH]

Stress: Forcibly exerted influence; pressure. Any condition or situation that causes strain or tension. Stress may be either physical or psychologic, or both. [NIH]

Subarachnoid: Situated or occurring between the arachnoid and the pia mater. [EU]

Supplementation: Adding nutrients to the diet. [NIH]

Support group: A group of people with similar disease who meet to discuss how better to cope with their cancer and treatment. [NIH]

Surfactant: A fat-containing protein in the respiratory passages which reduces the surface tension of pulmonary fluids and contributes to the elastic properties of pulmonary tissue. [NIH]

Therapeutics: The branch of medicine which is concerned with the treatment of diseases, palliative or curative. [NIH]

Thrombosis: The formation or presence of a blood clot inside a blood vessel. [NIH]

Ticks: Blood-sucking arachnids of the order Acarina. [NIH]

Tissue: A group or layer of cells that are alike in type and work together to perform a specific function. [NIH]

Topical: On the surface of the body. [NIH]

Toxic: Having to do with poison or something harmful to the body. Toxic substances usually cause unwanted side effects. [NIH]

Toxicity: The quality of being poisonous, especially the degree of virulence of a toxic microbe or of a poison. [EU]

Toxicology: The science concerned with the detection, chemical composition, and pharmacologic action of toxic substances or poisons and the treatment and prevention of toxic manifestations. [NIH]

Transfection: The uptake of naked or purified DNA into cells, usually eukaryotic. It is analogous to bacterial transformation. [NIH]

Ulcer: A localized necrotic lesion of the skin or a mucous surface. [NIH]

Ulceration: 1. The formation or development of an ulcer. 2. An ulcer. [EU]

Ulcerative colitis: Chronic inflammation of the colon that produces ulcers in its lining. This condition is marked by abdominal pain, cramps, and loose discharges of pus, blood, and mucus from the bowel. [NIH]

Unconscious: Experience which was once conscious, but was subsequently rejected, as the "personal unconscious". [NIH]

Uterus: The small, hollow, pear-shaped organ in a woman's pelvis. This is the organ in which a fetus develops. Also called the womb. [NIH]

Vaccines: Suspensions of killed or attenuated microorganisms (bacteria, viruses, fungi, protozoa, or rickettsiae), antigenic proteins derived from them, or synthetic constructs, administered for the prevention, amelioration, or treatment of infectious and other diseases. [NIH]

Vagina: The muscular canal extending from the uterus to the exterior of the body. Also called the birth canal. [NIH]

Vaginal: Of or having to do with the vagina, the birth canal. [NIH]

Venous: Of or pertaining to the veins. [EU]

Veterinary Medicine: The medical science concerned with the prevention, diagnosis, and treatment of diseases in animals. [NIH]

Vial: A small bottle. [EU]

Virus: Submicroscopic organism that causes infectious disease. In cancer therapy, some viruses may be made into vaccines that help the body build an immune response to, and kill, tumor cells. [NIH]

Vitamin A: A substance used in cancer prevention; it belongs to the family of drugs called retinoids. [NIH]

X-ray: High-energy radiation used in low doses to diagnose diseases and in high doses to treat cancer. [NIH]

INDEX

Printed in the United States
18634LVS00001B/13

9 780597 835872